Advance Praise

"Jenny provides the tips, tactics and game-changing approaches to anti-inflammatory eating that won't leave you feeling deprived. She makes breaking free from a bad diet super easy."

- Vani Hari
Creator of FoodBabe.com
New York Times Bestselling author of *The Food Babe Way*

"Inflammation creates and spreads disease, plain and simple. Jenny Carr's new masterpiece, *Peace of Cake*, is a FABULOUS resource that I will be sharing with all of my patients. How to swap out inflammatory ingredients that create disease with anti-inflammatory ingredients that create health and vibrancy?! Genius! Thank you, Jenny, for rocking it out! With this book, you will impact SO many lives!"

-Dr. Dana McGrady DOM, AP,
Author of Magnetic Soulpreneur
Physician, Better Health & Wellness Center

"Jenny Carr has blessed us with her extensive knowledge on inflammation. She distills a mass of information in a magnificent user friendly and inspired venue that gives us all a fine template from which to optimize our health and our quality of life. Her story of healing has been a courageous journey that I have personally witnessed and she is now a woman "on a mission"; a rejuvenated messenger, a true leader, tackling a big problem in our culture. As a nurse practitioner trained in nutritional biochemistry, I am excited about this book and consider it to be a phenomenal and critical tool for everyone who wants vibrant health in the context of a happy, meaningful and productive life."

- Laurie Shepherd Brown MSN, ANP-BC, CCN, BCC
Adult Nurse Practitioner - Board Certified
Certified Clinical Nutritionist
Integrative Health Consultant
Board Certified Life & Health Coach
Board Certified Executive & Leadership Coach
Founder, All Connected Life Coaching

"Great information for a population that desperately needs it."

- Dr. Stephan Siele DC, QN
Founder, Ascension Holistic Health Center

"You are what you eat – or perhaps more accurate is you are what your stomach absorbs, and this is something that I use in my clinical practice every day. Jenny Carr does a great job teaching the most important aspect of health using her own experience, science, and practical know-how, and that is your food intake. This book will teach you how to eat in the real world, and will can help you gain control of your health and start living instead of merely surviving. I recommend this book to anyone who is struggling with their health, doesn't know where to start with a diet, or needs parameters for health daily eating. It's a great addition to anyone's library and knowledge base. If you want to achieve and maintain optimal health, this is the book for you."

- Jason West DC NMD DCDBN FIAMA
Owner/Physician West Clinic
Author of the #1 Amazon bestsellers *Hidden Secrets to Curing Your Chronic Disease* & *Hidden Secrets to Daily Living*
Featured in *Doctored & Undoctored*, medical documentaries
Blogger – www.dailydosevitaminh.com

PEACE of Cake

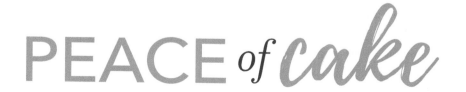

PEACE *of* *cake*

THE SECRET TO AN
ANTI-INFLAMMATORY DIET

JENNY CARR

NEW YORK

LONDON • NASHVILLE • MELBOURNE • VANCOUVER

PEACE of Cake

The Secret to an Anti-Inflammatory Diet

Published in New York, New York, by Morgan James Publishing in partnership with Difference Press. Morgan James is a trademark of Morgan James, LLC. www.MorganJamesPublishing.com

The Morgan James Speakers Group can bring authors to your live event. For more information or to book an event visit The Morgan James Speakers Group at www.TheMorganJamesSpeakersGroup.com.

ISBN 9781683509455 paperback
ISBN 9781683509462 eBook
Library of Congress Control Number: 2018931367

Cover Design by:
Megan Whitney
megan@creativeninjadesigns.com

Interior Design by:
Chris Treccani
www.3dogcreative.net

Photography by:
Jamye Chrisman Photography

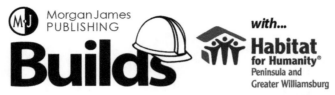

In an effort to support local communities, raise awareness and funds, Morgan James Publishing donates a percentage of all book sales for the life of each book to Habitat for Humanity Peninsula and Greater Williamsburg.

Get involved today! Visit
www.MorganJamesBuilds.com

To my mom and dad, who continue to walk beside me as we forge a path toward healing and vibrancy. Thank you for your unwavering support. And for Tosh, Chloe, and Brock. It is your love and encouragement at each step of my journey that have allowed this book to come to fruition. I am so grateful.

Table of Contents

Foreword

So many nutrition books are repeat information that it's rare when one of them really breaks out and teaches you something in a memorable way. This is one of those books. It's that good.

Jenny Carr came to my office as a patient in 2014. She had been studying overseas, and had become ravaged by a parasitic infection. I was fortunate to be one of the doctors who helped Jenny put her life back in order.

What sets Jenny apart is her ability to take control of and accept responsibility for her health. She walks her talk by not only writing about what she teaches, but living it. She beat the sugar addiction.

In these pages, you'll learn about the power of water, how your emotions affect your health, how to reprogram your triggers for unhealthy foods, and even how to *breathe.* You'll learn how to put your body back in harmony and balance by going to the very root of the problem, whether it's low energy, chronic fatigue syndrome, Lyme disease, fibromyalgia, or autoimmune conditions like rheumatoid arthritis, multiple sclerosis, Sjogren's, and lupus.

Hippocrates urges us, "Let food be thy medicine and medicine be thy food."

This cannot be overstated. We cannot overestimate the effect diet has on health. We have a saying in the office: "You are what you eat …

and if you are what you eat, are you fast, cheap, and easy?" Our fast and processed food culture has made it convenient and easy to get food that tastes good but has very little nutritional value. Worse, it can inflame us and compromise our health.

Peace of Cake is one of the best resources I've found for learning how to swap out unhealthy, inflammatory ingredients for healthy ones – and includes dozens of terrific recipes that walk the reader through how to do just that. You'll learn how to make everything from healthy pancakes and refreshing drinks to the titular cake.

This book is a wonderful and much-needed information source for people struggling with both serious health conditions and people who just want more energy. I'm recommending it to all of my patients. I believe that once you read it you'll be as big a fan of Jenny Carr as I am.

Jason West DC NMD DCDBN FIAMA
Owner/Physician West Clinic
Author of the Amazon best-sellers
Hidden Secrets to Curing Your Chronic Disease
& Hidden Secrets to Daily Living
Blogger at www.dailydosevitaminh.com

Introduction

"Let food be thy medicine and medicine be thy food."
Hippocrates

I'm guessing you've tried an anti-inflammatory diet. If nothing else, you've likely tried bits and pieces of an anti-inflammatory diet. It seemed to help, but falling off the wagon was inevitable, and hopping back on was much more difficult than you anticipated. You know it could have had huge impact on your life, yet the protocol makes you feel deprived, and sticking with all of the rules of anti-inflammatory eating is totally overwhelming. Where do you even begin?

Peace Of Cake was written from me to you. It is for those willing to raise their game of self-care, but need a simplified process to do so. You know you need to eliminate inflammation from your body, yet you also want to be able to enjoy your favorite comfort foods, socialize with your friends, and indulge in celebrations. You are looking for *lasting* change in a way that is manageable and *fun*.

Peace Of Cake is the secret to maintaining anti-inflammatory eating. By eliminating one main ingredient and swapping it out for a non-inflammatory alternative, many of the other top inflammatory foods fall to the wayside, creating a more effective and streamlined method for eating in a way that supports your body.

Because you are reading this book, my guess is that chronic inflammation *is* stacking up in your body, and you know something needs to change. You might be experiencing subtle discomfort. It's possible the discomfort has turned into a bigger issue. Your body is yelling at you to get the inflammation out. You know following an anti-inflammatory diet can make all the difference, but the gap between knowledge and action seems too great.

The truth is, we all show up to anti-inflammatory eating in our own perfect timing. Typically, we turn toward these lifestyle changes when we have hit rock bottom, and the inflammation in our body is causing us to miss out on the life we envisioned for ourselves.

My rock bottom came in 2009 after I had my first child and felt like I was losing my identity entirely. Once a Division One cross-country ski racer, marathon runner, and overall adventurer, I had gained 55 pounds from my pregnancy and the weight was not coming off. I wanted to exercise more, but I was too exhausted from basic day-to-day chores. In fact, I found myself in bed by 7 pm most nights. Nausea and bloat became the norm. Instead of bouncing back to the athlete and supermom that I had planned on being, I was struggling to accomplish the simple tasks of living and raising my baby boy. To be honest, shame permeated each cell within me. I compared myself to all of my peers who *appeared* to be bouncing back from their pregnancies just fine. This exacerbated my shame. I wanted to go into hiding.

My commitment to anti-inflammatory eating was prompted not so much by a desire to eliminate my symptoms, but rather to gain back my identity. I needed to find *me*. I needed to be able to run and ski, to throw dinner parties and enjoy life. All of those things in my life were quickly slipping away.

Many people who I work with are looking for a life of freedom. A life that allows them to play with their children and grandchildren free of pain. A life that allows them to step up and be the athletes they always dreamed of. A life that allows them to enjoy social events without having to track down every bathroom within the building because of an upset stomach.

A life that affords them the energy and clear thinking to start their own businesses and thrive as entrepreneurs. If you are like me, you are looking for the freedom to be a mom, wife, and friend who is dependable and reliable. No more energy crashes, spinning mind, or painful muscles that put you in bed for days at a time.

Inflammation shows up differently for each of us. It targets the areas that are most susceptible in our bodies. Because we are all unique, it is helpful to take some time to figure out how inflammation is affecting you. When we connect the symptoms we are experiencing with inflammation and then determine exactly how that is impacting our overall ability to live life to the fullest, a powerful and more sincere motivation emerges to maintain anti-inflammatory eating.

Believe me, once you experience the contrast of how you feel after removing inflammation from your body, you will not want to go back to your old habits. We are all walking around feeling sub-par, oftentimes without even knowing it. If you are reading this book, it is because you have been led here to gain health and grow young. This book holds the key to regeneration and vibrant living. Are you ready to take the next step?

Anti-inflammatory eating will have you feeling *amazing*, physically. And, there is a bonus side effect that, in my opinion, trumps everything else we have spoken of thus far. It is the gift of feeling grounded and experiencing true joy in life both mentally and emotionally.

A perfect example of this transformation is from one of my clients, Joe. Joe came to me with two goals. He wanted to lose weight, but most importantly, he was looking to alleviate back pain from a herniated disc. Surgery had been discussed. He knew following an anti-inflammatory diet would help him lose weight, and he was pretty sure it would help with the pain. Joe traveled a lot for work and was newly married. The stress of his work showed up as anger in his marriage.

As Joe shifted his diet, he did lose weight and eliminate back pain. But more importantly to Joe, he discovered an increase of energy, and the dissipation of anger. As he continued to eat clean, his relationships continued to improve. While following this diet did not give him more time off from the road or remove the stress of travel, it did give him the energy to do his job and work at his marriage. Now 50 pounds lighter and free of back pain and anger, Joe lives a more joyful life with his beautiful wife and three amazing kids.

Inflammation showed up in the form of back pain, weight gain, low energy, and anger for Joe. In my case, I experienced digestive disorders, depression, fatigue, weight gain, and low-grade body aches. The differences in response are because inflammation targets the areas where we each are most vulnerable. Another example of inflammation showing up uniquely for each person was with my son Tosh. During Tosh's first year of life, he was constantly sick. He had chronic ear and throat infections that turned into abscesses and threatened his life during two terrifying events. While I did not know it at the time, Tosh's health issues showed up in his body from chronic inflammation. The inflammation suppressed his immune system so much that as soon as he got a whiff of the common cold, he would be knocked down for weeks with high fevers and infections. We spent months in and out of hospitals, some of that time being in the ICU.

It was amazing to see the shift in Tosh's health once I changed his diet to 100 percent anti-inflammatory foods. He began to heal with incredible speed. I remember the day when Tosh got a cold without it leading to a super high fever and a visit to the hospital. I was *so* excited that my son was finally healthy enough to simply get a cold, and have it be just that. Seven years later, Tosh continues to eat an anti-inflammatory diet. He has never been back to the hospital, and I cannot remember a time he has needed antibiotics since changing the way he eats.

More than likely, inflammation is affecting you in more ways than you realize. In fact, chronic inflammation is the root cause of most ailments, conditions, and dis-ease, and has been reported to be the underlying cause of death for seven out of ten people in the United States. While there may be additional factors contributing to our health issues, such as genetic make-up, structural injuries, or unwanted inhabitants living within our organs, we have the ability to eliminate *much* of the inflammation in our body through diet. This relieves our immune system and allows the cells within us to regenerate.

The trick to healing is to ensure we do not numb out our symptoms. Our society is generally in the habit of taking pain medication, high blood pressure medication, allergy medication, or Pepto-Bismol-like products (to mention only a few) in order to suppress our symptoms. The problem is that by doing so, we interfering with our body's ability to speak loudly and clearly to us. We are meant to experience vitality and health. If we are not, it simply means there are opportunities to heal our symptoms through change rather than continue to cover them up. One of the greatest assets I have gained in this life is the ability to truly listen to my body and adjust my actions accordingly. I wish the same for you.

Eating an anti-inflammatory diet is the foundation of healing. Without it, healing takes a *much* longer time, and sometimes isn't possible at all. Eating an anti-inflammatory diet, in fact, has the ability to catapult you into health without any complementary medical treatments. Truth be told, 98 percent of my clients have healed their ailments, conditions, and dis-ease by simply swapping out inflammatory foods for options that do not inflame, while adopting a lifestyle to support the body's ability to heal such as drinking sufficient water, gently moving the body, getting good rest, and becoming mindful of their thinking. With that said, one more bonus of eating this way is that if you choose to use complementary medicine to help you heal, the treatments are generally ten times more potent and effective.

A simple shift to anti-inflammatory eating has led my clients into the lives of their dreams: lives of confidence, empowerment, freedom, energy, and vitality. Lives free of pain and dis-ease. I have helped clients reverse their autoimmune conditions, massively reduce (or eradicate) joint pain, support the healing of digestive conditions, lower blood pressure, reduce insulin for type 1 diabetes and reverse type 2 diabetes, clear up skin conditions, eliminate asthma, clear brain fog, reverse depression, improve headaches, support the balance of hormones, improve athletic performance, and lose unwanted weight. This is a *short* list of what can be accomplished by adopting an anti-inflammatory diet.

Throughout this book, you will learn the top six inflammatory foods and how to swap them out. In particular, you will learn the trick to swapping out processed sugar for naturally occurring sugars that don't trigger inflammation. I will share with you my methods to support the detox process as you remove stagnant and chronic inflammation from your body. In addition, I will teach you methods to streamline your cooking so you can stick to this method of eating with ease. We'll learn the difference between regular protein and clean protein, along with approximately how many grams to eat each day. You will learn how drinking enough clean water each day is arguably the most potent method of removing inflammation from your body. You will become empowered as you learn how to stop cravings in their tracks. This book is a compilation of my knowledge, training, and experience, designed to give you the best bang for your buck when it comes to removing inflammation from your body. Each chapter was chosen from among the topics that consistently propel my clients into vibrant living.

Remember, most people fall short in the gap between knowledge and action. As you read this book, I encourage you to take action. Don't wait for tomorrow. It's time for you to be the change *you wish* to see in *your* world. As you take action, be sure to check out Part 2 of this book, chock-full of delicious and comforting anti-inflammatory recipes like pizza, cookies, pancakes, and muffins!

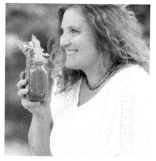 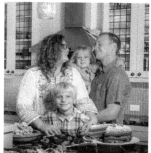 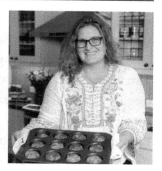

Chapter 1

My Story

*"Two roads diverged in a wood, and I - I took the one less traveled by.
And that has made all the difference."*
Robert Frost

How Anti-Inflammatory Living Helped Save My Life

I came to anti-inflammatory eating to regain and re-define my identity. I had gained a lot of extra weight, was exhausted, had digestive issues, and – overall – felt depressed. After following through with an anti-inflammatory diet, those symptoms literally melted away. I lost all of the excess weight, was able to start exercising again, and accomplished a ton at home and work because my energy level soared. Most significantly to me, I found joy around every corner of life. Pretty amazing what eating this way can do for us!

While I did not know it at the time, all of that practice maintaining anti-inflammatory eating was preparation for the biggest battle of my life. Three years ago, I was diagnosed with a severe parasite infection whose origins went back 20 years to a trip I'd taken to Africa. The infection was further complicated by backpacking around Southeast Asia, the South Pacific, two fishing trips to the Amazon, and multiple trips to South America. I have always considered myself an adventurer, and never once during my travels did I think, *Careful what you do, you might get parasites!*

Parasites are tricky and can do a lot of unseen and unfelt damage. In my case, by the time I was diagnosed, the parasites had put actual holes in my organs and had eaten away some of my endocrine glands. This actually prompted my body to go into organ failure at one point! But as much damage as these river monsters wreaked as they took over my body, the neurotoxins they released were even worse. They literally poisoned me, paralyzing my legs, preventing me from speaking, causing me to spin with vertigo like a drunken sailor for weeks at a time. All of this meant that I was no longer a functioning mom, wife, friend, and coach. I was literally trying to stay alive – a prisoner of my own bed.

As these parasites died off, they released horrific bacteria and viruses, some that were life-threatening, others that created an autoimmune condition. At one point, I had four different strains of Lyme dis-ease: Leptospira, Borellia, Bartonella, and Babesia.

It felt like the weight of the world was on me, and my prognosis was not good. The parasites and Lyme had made their way into my brain stem, my spinal cord, and deep within my organs and glands. And there was this horrifying math: adult parasites can lay up to 5000 eggs per day, and bacteria is constantly dividing and reproducing at lightning speed. My body simply couldn't keep up. My immune system was beyond compromised, my liver and kidneys were in massive overload, and all the while, the bugs causing this continued to exist and replicate. I felt completely defeated much of the time.

There was approximately a year during this three-year period of extreme illness when I was operating off only 1 to 2 percent of the energy that should have been available to me. When I say operating, I mean surviving. I was bedridden, most days. Often, the toxins were so intense that it felt as though I had drunk a gallon of bleach. I would lie in bed for days at a time, holding onto the sheet for dear life because I had the spins so bad I felt as though I was going to fall out onto the floor. I had to army crawl to get to the toilet, and was completely unable to eat. My breathing was heavily labored, and sometimes I could not get my legs or muscles to move. Words would form in my brain, yet when I tried to speak, nothing would come out. I could remember very little. I was scared for my life, and rightfully so.

I worked with a number of complementary doctors and health practitioners. While all of the treatments they prescribed were essential to my recovery, so was eating an anti-inflammatory diet. In fact, I believe that following an anti-inflammatory diet and lifestyle played a major role in saving my life. *If* I had not been following a strict anti-inflammatory diet (when I was able to eat), *if* I had not been drinking a gallon of water each day to push out as many toxins as possible, *if* I had not been practicing breathing to calm down my nervous system, I would simply not have had enough energy to keep me alive.

I was told that, at minimum, it would likely take a couple of years to heal. While I cannot say that I am 100 percent healed at this point, I am well on my way to vibrant, healthy living. I feel amazing! Once again, I get to be the mom, friend, wife, daughter, and coach that I was meant to show up as in this life.

It has been three years since I found out about the parasites, but only eight months since I was diagnosed with Lyme. The rate of my healing is operating at lightning speed, especially for someone who likely went undiagnosed with Lyme for 20 years. In my experience, people who follow an anti-inflammatory diet typically have a tenfold return on the effectiveness of the complementary medicine that they choose to help them heal. I've seen this phenomenon over and over again. It is truly magical.

I want you to know that I have walked your path, in more ways than one. I have been the new mom who felt as though her identity was gone. I have been the woman who had underlying chronic symptoms that continued to build up and slowly affected the quality of my life, including depression. I have gone from athlete, to not … and back again. I have gone through two pregnancies: one eating an anti-inflammatory diet, and the other giving in to typical pregnancy cravings. (These pregnancies were drastically different in how I felt on many levels.)

I have been diagnosed with an autoimmune dis-ease. I have nearly died from strange and bizarre parasitic infections. I have felt the incredible mental and emotional well-being that come from following an anti-inflammatory lifestyle. Most of all, I have been the mom who, under all conditions, maintained an anti-inflammatory eating practice. With two kids, my own business, and major health issues, I figured out how to make anti-inflammatory living a reality for me. It's not always pretty. I don't serve new and creative dishes at each meal. I keep things super simple so that I can be in integrity and walk my talk. But this has literally saved my life, and I know it can have a similar impact on you.

Perspective is everything. Our struggles only help us to savor the beauty in life more intensely. They allow us to grow and learn from the unhealthy stories we tell ourselves. What a journey of growth, of healing, and of gaining perspective I have had the honor of experiencing.

Chapter 2

H2O, Not to Be Underestimated

"Success is the sum of small efforts, repeated day in and day out."
Robert Collier

Jump Start the Elimination of Inflammation Without Changing Your Diet

How many of you have told yourself that you will start a diet right *after* girls night out, or *after* the Ben & Jerry's pint is empty, or *after* your friend's wedding? You can fill in the words following *after* with any life obstacle, celebration, or event. That's where we create all of these rules about when and how change happens. Beyond the rules that we set for ourselves, it can be difficult to know where *your* entry point is for following an anti-inflammatory diet. Do you take sugar out of your diet first, maybe dairy? Then again... the whole gluten-free thing is something worth looking into. I have the perfect answer for you. It's

5

perfect because it does not involve food and you can begin right this very minute.

Drinking *enough* water is a *key* component in removing inflammation from your body. And it's perfect. You don't need to go to the grocery store, or swap out foods to start, yet it makes the most profound difference. Even better, all you need is a water bottle or glass to begin; right here, right now.

I know you *know* about the importance of drinking water. If fact, everyone I have ever spoken to in regards to health knows the importance of hydration, yet very few people truly understand the critical role water plays in eliminating inflammation from the body. To be honest, if you walk away with nothing else from this book, promise me you will follow through with the single action step laid out in this chapter. Even if you do not change your diet, I can promise you that adding significant water to your day may be the single most powerful tool you can use on your journey to healing.

One of the first questions that I ask my clients during their initial consult is, "How much water do you drink?" The answer I most frequently get is, "Very little, but I'm just not thirsty." I love this answer because it opens up space for a very interesting science experiment, and science experiments are my favorite! I love them because it's one thing for someone to tell you what to do. It is entirely different when you allow your body to speak to you, and *experience* how your daily actions affect it. Truly, this is the gift I wish to bestow upon each and every one of you.

I have always been a big believer in explaining the *why* for doing something. So while you will experience your body speaking to you with our little science experiment, allow me to explain the why behind you not feeling thirsty, even when drinking a minimal amount of water. From an evolutionary standpoint, we have a thirst mechanism that can be turned on or shut off. When we were hunters and gatherers, we would walk for hours and many times even a day or two, moving from one water source to the next. Often there would be very little water available to drink during these migrations. In order to stop the physical discomfort thirst brings about, the thirst mechanism would be deactivated. This happened naturally whenever the body realized water was not available for it to drink. Instead of spending days feeling the suffering sensation thirst brings upon us, our body simply deactivates the thirst mechanism, a default response that continues unabated the less water we drink. Likewise, if we start the morning drinking lots of water, it creates a signal saying a source of water is near us and available. This in turn *activates* your thirst mechanism, creating a sensation of *more* thirst as the amount of water you drink increases. This is your body's way of talking to you, saying, "Yes please! If water is available, I want *more* of it!" But don't take my word, let me lay out a little science experiment for you to see how your body chooses to speak with you.

The goal of this experiment is to drink one gallon of water per day, for all adult-sized humans. I know, that sounds like a staggering amount. Hang with me for one week, and then make your decision. What you will likely find is a significant reduction in inflammation, the number on your scale dropping, less stiffness in your joints, a mental feeling of grounded-ness, and likely fewer cravings. Sound good? If so, here's the easiest way to accomplish drinking that gallon of water each day.

The first thing you want to do is get a large water bottle, preferably one quart or 32 ounces. (You will be drinking four 32-ounce water bottles throughout the day.) When you wake up in the morning, go to the bathroom, weigh yourself (don't worry, it's fun because you can watch the inflammation melt off), and then chug the water bottle. For some, channeling their inner college-beer-drinking self helps bring them back to how easy chugging the water actually can be. If that was never you, no worries. Simply take your water and throw it down the hatch. The truth is, if you *focus* on drinking your water quickly and efficiently – in one sitting – you will make it happen. It only takes about 52 seconds to drink an entire quart of water if that is all you are doing.

The problem for most people is that they pour themselves a glass of water or a cup of tea/coffee in the morning. They begin to check emails and Facebook, pack their kids' lunches, and get dressed. Halfway through their water (if they are lucky enough to get themselves a glass of water before the coffee and tea), it's time to leave for the day. Because of all the distractions, their water was never drunk, or at least not much of it. This automatically sends a message to the body, telling it to keep the thirst mechanism low, not much water is available today.

If instead, you stand in one place and drink your quart of water *before* you do anything else other than use the restroom and weigh yourself, your body thinks you have a huge source of water available to you, and you actually become thirstier the more water you drink. It's such a fun experiment! Once you have the morning chug down, you will want to immediately fill up your water bottle again.

Have you ever been thirsty with an empty cup sitting right in front of you, but while you wanted to drink, you didn't because of the effort required to get up and fill up your glass? If you're like 99 percent of us, the answer is: yes. So let's avoid that happening by filling up your water bottle right away.

The next goal is to drink your second quart of water by lunch. Ideally, you drink water from your second water bottle between breakfast and lunch. Around noon, or when you stop for lunch, the idea is to chug any water left from water bottle two. Repeat for water bottle number three, chugging any remnants at 3 in the afternoon, with the last water bottle going down the hatch by 6 pm. I encourage finishing off your last quart of water by six so that you have time to use the bathroom enough before going to bed. That way you won't wake up as frequently to use the bathroom at night.

Speaking of the bathroom ... I know what you're thinking. "I'm going to have to pee every two seconds!" Truth be told, you will have to pee quite a bit the first couple of weeks that you implement this science experiment. The reason is because you are pushing crazy amounts of inflammation (or toxins) out of your body and into your bladder. Imagine your bladder as if it were an empty pond. As the inflammation and toxins are pushed out of your body, they condense in your bladder. As you can imagine, sitting in a pool of toxins is no fun, so the bladder sends a signal to your brain sharing the need to eliminate the condensed toxins ASAP. What you will find is that you frequently will need to pee, but the elimination will likely be quite short. This is because while there may not be a ton of fluid in your bladder once it signals the need to eliminate, there are a ton of toxins. As you continue with your consistent water drinking, you will find that the built-up chronic inflammation begins to disperse, lowering the concentration of toxins in your bladder and allowing your body to hydrate as it is meant to. How does this help you? Within a few weeks of time, you will be peeing much less often, and your elimination will be more thorough and take time. This is a good sign that significant inflammation has left your body!

Why is all of this water drinking so important? Peeing and sweating are the two major ways people eliminate inflammation from their bodies. There are other methods, but these are the major ways to be efficient at the elimination of inflammation. And while we cannot sweat all day long, we can drink water and pee all day long. Water is to your liver and kidneys what gasoline is to a car. If your car is running on empty, or if it has poor-quality gasoline going in, it will slowly sputter down the road. However, if your car is on full and has high-quality gasoline, you will have no problem zipping down the road to your desired destination. The same is true of water. If you drink enough clean water (one gallon per day for the purpose of eliminating inflammation from the body), your liver will have superpower abilities to process the built-up toxins and inflammation residing within you that can cause a host of major issues if not flushed out.

If the liver and kidney do not have enough clean water, they cannot process all of the toxins being added to the body, so toxins are reabsorbed. From here, one of two things happens. Option one: the toxins are directly reabsorbed back into your organs. When this happens, you can become quite ill, quickly. The second possibility is that the body will create a storage space for these toxins by pushing them as far away from the organs as possible in pockets of fat tissues. If there is a large overload of toxins being reabsorbed in the body, you will experience an increase in body fat because the body is literally creating more fat to store the toxins in. It is a survival mechanism to push the toxins as far away from the organs as possible.

Importantly to note, many of my clients lose 2-10 pounds in the first week of working with me (even if they're not really looking to drop weight), simply because they are finally fueling their liver, which is allowing toxins and inflammation to be pushed out of their body through water consumption. I absolutely love watching this transformation take place. Not only does the number on the scale typically decrease, but people start to notice how much better they feel. One of the top benefits of increasing water intake to a gallon per day is the exponential increase in energy that people feel. Along with that increase in energy, people will often find that their digestion begins to work more smoothly, their joints experience more mobility, their skin clears up, and they sleep better at night. In fact, one of my clients just recently wrote to me saying that after one week of drinking a gallon of water per day, her gut is finally working and regularity has come back for the first time in months. All of this simply by increasing the amount of water you drink. Pretty cool, right?

Some people question the amount of water I encourage them to drink. But imagine your body as a dried-out riverbed. In that riverbed are many rocks and pebbles, representing the toxins and inflammation sitting in your body. Now, let's imagine a slow and steady trickle of water beginning to run down the riverbed. The water will push out *some* sand and small pebbles, but we are looking to push out large quantities of stones and boulders. The goal is not to simply stay alive by eliminating small amounts of inflammation, but to thrive by getting rid of the smoldering chronic inflammation. So now imagine a torrential downpour; the riverbed fills up entirely. Soon, the pebbles, stones, and boulders are pushed downstream and out of the riverbed. This is the same concept for your body. It's one thing to be hydrated; it's a whole new level to use the consumption of clean water as a tool to eliminate inflammation from your body.

So while the peeing may be obnoxious for a few days, think of pivoting your thoughts ever so slightly. Instead of predetermining its annoyance, remember that peeing and sweating are the two primary methods for eliminating both inflammation and fat from the body. So embrace the peeing. Know that through this simple step, you are making tremendous headway in gaining health and eliminating inflammation from your body.

Now go find yourself a quart of water and give it a good chug.

Chapter 3

The Secret Recipe

"A thousand disappointments from the past cannot equal the power of one positive action right now."
Ralph Marston

Swap Out One Inflammatory Food to Melt Away Inflammation

When I started my anti-inflammatory eating journey, I learned what the top inflammatory foods were that significantly impact people. These are the foods that I can make a blanket statement about in regards to their effect on inflammation in your body. These top inflammatory foods are processed sugar, processed wheat, cow dairy, inflammatory oils, genetically modified foods (otherwise known as GMOs), and alcohol. Yes, I always save alcohol for the last, as I know that can be a tough one! Of course there are other inflammatory "foods" such as preservatives, additives, pesticides, etc.; however, I find that when you eliminate the top six inflammatory foods and purchase organic fruits and vegetables, you pretty much eliminate all the other preservatives, pesticides, and chemicals that one may find hiding in packaged food.

While there may be other foods potentially inflaming you, it's nearly impossible to positively identify them until you have removed the major six players adding to chronic inflammation. Many times people will come to me for a first session and explain that they are sensitive to broccoli, carrots, and peas (just as an example), yet they are eating a diet packed full of processed sugar and inflammatory oils. Unless you are truly allergic to a food, meaning you have an allergic reaction likely requiring some form of medication to quickly reverse the symptoms, it is difficult to know what additional foods are truly inflaming you. With that said, it is very possible that peas could be inflaming you, and in order to find out, you want to remove these top major contributors of inflammation for at least two weeks *and then* see how your body responds to eating peas. One of the beautiful aspects of eating an anti-inflammatory diet is that food allergies often disappear over time. These allergies are often caused by leaky gut, and anti-inflammatory eating has great success in helping to reverse that.

I was recently speaking to a client whom I'll call Deb. When we started working together a little less than a year ago, she told me that she was unable to eat raw vegetables, and that when she tried, they went straight through her and she would have to look for the nearest bathroom very quickly. If this describes you, you know how it affects your freedom in life. You know where every public restroom is in your town and plan social events according to how you are feeling and what is available to eat. Deb ate a pretty healthy diet before we started working together, but by swapping out a few of the top inflammatory foods and identifying what inflamed her on an individual basis, she is now able to eat all of the raw veggies she wants! No more dashes to the bathroom. She finally can experience the freedom to do what she wants, when she wants. She is in control, and you can be, too.

I know you want freedom from inflammation, and freedom from your symptoms. And, it is possible. It is possible without drugs and doctor visits. As you fuel your body with the food it is intended to eat, the cells that reside within actually begin to regenerate. It is a scientific fact that cells either regenerate or degenerate. There's no holding steady and staying the same, contrary to my belief for years. When we remove chronic inflammation, fuel the cells with real nutrition, provide enough water to the body, allow ourselves adequate rest, and move our muscles, the cells within your body magically begin to *regenerate*. This literally means you can grow young.

At the age of 65, Sally thought she was too old to lose weight and get healthy. Over the years, she had tried many different "diets," each a temporary fix. Yet within a few months of adopting an anti-inflammatory diet, her beliefs of being too old to accomplish her goals were shattered. She lost 50 pounds by following this process and was able to get off all of her medications, including high blood pressure meds.

Sally is one example of many who have grown young following this anti-inflammatory eating lifestyle. How would it feel to get off of medication? How would it feel to lose unwanted weight and move your body in ways it has not moved for years? More importantly, how would it feel to experience this without feeling deprived and overwhelmed?

My guess is that the idea of removing processed sugar, modern-day wheat, cow dairy, inflammatory oils, GMOs, and alcohol sounds far from easy. In fact, my guess is that it sounds downright overwhelming to you, not to mention depriving. I understand those emotions to the core. Trying to go out to eat and telling the server all that I cannot eat often felt like I was in a jail cell. Reminding myself of the top six inflammatory foods that I was to stay away from, especially at first, felt like a memory game in and of itself. But because I have walked my talk and eaten an anti-inflammatory diet for nearly a decade while coaching many beautiful clients as they shifted into a state of health through diet and lifestyle, I've been able to identify the number one biggest player affecting most of the inflammation in your body right now.

By removing this single, top inflammatory food and swapping it out with something that tastes similar yet regenerates, rather than degenerates, your cells, you can begin to lose weight, reverse adverse health conditions, up your athletic game, experience a sensation of peace and grounded-ness, and ultimately experience high levels of joy in your life.

By now you must be wondering what this top secret and highly inflammatory food is. It is a food that was labeled by the FDA, a number of years ago, as toxic. This is the FDA speaking, which in my experience has been quite reserved about making bold statements such as this over the years. This food has been directly linked to types 1 and 2 diabetes, heart dis-ease, tooth decay, cancer, fatty liver, and Alzheimer's. There is scientific evidence that this food contributes to these specific conditions, but beyond that, we must remember that it is the number one most inflammatory ingredient out there, which means it often rests at the root of much dis-ease in the body. There are over 50 names for this highly inflammatory food, making it quite challenging for the consumer to avoid. To top it off, it is hands-down the most addictive food available to us. You guessed it: sugar. And not just any sugar, but processed sugar.

56 NAMES FOR PROCESSED SUGAR

Barley malt	Dehydrated cane juice	Golden sugar	Molasses
Barbados sugar	Demerara sugar	Golden syrup	Muscovado
Beet sugar	Dextran	Grape sugar	Panocha
Brown sugar	Dextrose	High fructose corn syrup	Powdered sugar
Buttered syrup	Diastatic malt	Honey (unless it's raw)	Yellow sugar
Cane juice	Diastase	Icing sugar	Refiner's syrup
Cane sugar	Ethyl maltol	Invert sugar	Rice syrup
Caramel	Free flowing brown sugars	Lactose	Sorbitol
Corn syrup	Fructose	Malt	Sorghum syrup
Corn syrup solids	Fruit juice	Maltodextrin	Sucrose
Confectioner's sugar	Fruit juice concentrate	Maltose	Sugar (granulated)
Carob syrup	Galactose	Malt syrup	Treacle
Caster sugar	Glucose	Mannitol	Turbinado sugar
Date sugar	Glucose solids		

Processed sugar hides in everything! According to endocrinologist Dr. Robert Lustig, processed sugar is in 74 percent of the foods in every grocery store. While we all know when we are eating obvious sugars such as cakes, cookies, and doughnuts, it's the hidden sugar that can get the best of us.

My challenge to you is to become a renegade researcher for the next two weeks. Read the label on every food you put into your mouth. If there is processed sugar in it, either opt out or swap it out for a food that uses raw honey, pure maple syrup, raw agave, liquid stevia, or unrefined coconut sugar. For the agave and honey, it's important that it is *raw*, meaning that it's never been heated or processed. Raw honey, in particular, has incredible anti-bacterial and anti-microbial properties. It is believed to help alleviate allergies and is full of vitamins and minerals. However, when raw honey is heated, it changes the honey on a molecular level and creates inflammation. The same is true of agave when it is processed. It is quite rare to find raw agave in packaged products.

Beyond these concentrated sweeteners, it is important to know that whole fruit provides you with an array of vitamins, minerals, and anti-oxidants that support the healing of the body. As long as you are eating the *whole fruit*, rather than the fruit juice, the sugar you consume from items like bananas, oranges, apples, berries, pears, etc. has incredible potency to support living vibrantly. As soon as you remove the fiber and pulp from a fruit, then the sugar can create some level of inflammation.

If you're interested to know more about the direct correlation between health and the consumption of processed sugar, check out this timeline below. It demonstrates an indisputable connection between dis-ease in the body and sugar consumption.

8,000 BC – It is estimated that sugar cane was first domesticated in New Guinea and then spread to China and beyond.

350 AD – Sugarcane growers in India discover and master how to crystallize sugar using a boiling process of refining cane juice.

11ᵗʰ Century to 1700 – Cane sugar is referred to as the white gold, costing upwards of today's equivalent of $50/pound and making it unattainable for anyone other than the noble and rich.

1747 – Sugar beets are identified as a new source of commercial sugar, which drives down the prices and makes sugar more affordable to the middle and lower classes. Because of the low cost, sugar is now added to candy, tea, coffee, and many other food items.

1800 – A French medical student identifies the first group of patients with rheumatoid arthritis, a condition in which the body's own immune system attacks the joint lining and cartilage. (Two centuries later, medical research will link sugar as a cause for rheumatoid arthritis.)

1900 – The average British citizen now eats about 100 pounds of sugar per year, and the average American eats approximately 40 pounds a year.

1906 – A German physician, Dr. Alzheimer, first identifies a form of dementia. By the end of the 20th century, an estimated five million Americans will be diagnosed with Alzheimer's dis-ease each year.

1910 – A medical explanation emerges in the US for the rising rates of diabetes: the pancreas of a diabetic patient was unable to produce insulin, a chemical the body uses to break down sugar.

1962 – An estimated 13 percent of American adults meet the criteria for obesity.

1967 – A Japanese scientist invents a cost-effective industrial process for using enzymes to convert glucose in cornstarch to fructose. High-fructose corn syrup derived from corn becomes a cheap alternative sweetener to beet and sugarcane sugar.

1975 – In the US, 400 new cases of cancer occur for every 100,000 people, or a total of 864,000 people each year.

1984 – Soft drinks companies such as Pepsi and Coca-Cola switch from sugar to the cheaper high-fructose corn syrup in US production facilities.

1992 – Cancer rates have climbed to 510 cases for every 100,000 people in the US.

2004 – Obesity now affects 24.5 percent of US adults.

2005 – Each US citizen now eats about 100 pounds of added sugars each year, up from approximately 40 pounds in 1900.

2008 – The average American eats 37.8 pounds of high-fructose corn syrup every year, mostly unknowingly because it is laced in thousands of processed food and drink products.

2008 – Obesity rates hit an all-time high of 32 percent for men and 35 percent for women. Obesity is considered a factor in nearly 400,000 deaths per year.

2011 – The United Nations declares that non-communicable dis-eases – diabetes, cancer, chronic respiratory and cardiovascular dis-ease – have overtaken infectious dis-eases as the world's leading cause of death.

2015 – The World Health Organization releases official guidelines on sugar intake. They recommend that free sugars (essentially sugars *other* than naturally occurring sugars in whole foods like fruit) make up no more than 10 percent of our daily diet, with a further suggestion to limit them to 5 percent. Applauded by scientists and nutritionists worldwide and criticized by industry, it's the most progressive move to date.

Information collected from: http://hippocratesinst.org/the-sugar-timeline and http://sugarcoateddoc.com/sugar-timeline/

If you Google this topic and dig a bit further, you will find loads of interesting information about the timing of the introduction of processed sugar and the negative effects of sugar intake. In addition, you will see the battle between the FDA and Big Sugar corporations who have worked at trying to convince the general public that sugar is a nutritional component that should be added to everyone's diet as a way to keep one's weight in check (statement made in 1975).

When you look at this timeline, do you see any similarity to that of tobacco? A parallel of encouraging people to use tobacco, followed by statements that it causes cancer? Through work such as Dr. Robert Lustig's studies, sugar is beginning to be defined as a drug – as a poison connected to an array of health conditions causing death and overall suffering in life.

Someone could argue that it's not sugar creating such havoc in the general public's health. And I agree that there are other contributing factors such as dehydration, stress, lack of sleep, and environmental toxins. But facts are facts. Whether you want to read more into the timeline or not, listen to Dr. Robert Lustig's keynote presentation *Sugar: The Bitter Truth*. (Dr. Lustig is a pediatric endocrinologist at the University of California in San Francisco and a leading expert on the effects of sugar in human physiology.) Or you could try something more personal, like one of my favorite science experiments on yourself. You will come to find the truth.

Sugar is frequently at the root of inflammation, and inflammation is at the root of nearly every adverse health condition.

So many of us don't realize how bad we feel! We might wake up with some nausea, but over time, it just becomes a pattern. Within a few months, that nausea is the new norm and a few months later, we don't remember what it felt like to wake up without nausea. The same is true of any chronic symptom. If it is low-grade and persistent, chronic illness becomes the new norm. Very often my clients tell me that they didn't realize they could feel this good once they have adopted and maintained an anti-inflammatory diet. It is one of the greatest surprises in life, and is in perfect alignment with Kevin Trudeau's famous quote, "Most people have no idea how good their body is designed to feel." My challenge to you: take that bold step and allow yourself to feel all of the goodness by swapping out processed sugar.

In removing processed sugar from your diet, many of the top inflammatory foods will also fall to the wayside by default. This secret to eating an anti-inflammatory diet makes it so much more manageable. By removing processed sugar, you automatically eliminate 99% of the alcohol, processed wheat, and cow dairy in your diet. In addition, you end up removing a significant amount of inflammatory oils and GMOs. It's my magic trick. Beyond magically eliminating many of these inflammatory foods by swapping out processed sugar for sweet treats that do not inflame, the removal of processed sugar alone has the power to heal many people's health conditions.

The trick is to read those labels. Focus primarily on removing processed sugar and swapping it out with sugars that support your body. As you eat some of the tasty treats provided in Part 2 of this book, try on the grocery store food swaps, or simply use the approved non-inflammatory sugars, all while drinking your water (can't forget that important step), your body will begin to feel the best it has in years – possibly ever!

Heather, a sugar-holic, came to me asking for help. She told me that she simply could not continue living the way she was. She felt out of her mind and totally ungrounded. A mother of three young kids, she was constantly on the go, and while she had put forth worthy effort in the past, she could not figure out how to *maintain* anti-inflammatory eating. She had chronic knee pain, headaches, rashes, and anxiety. Life was not feeling amazing for Heather, and she had to do something about it. By following the steps in this book, after two weeks, she said she no longer had a craving to indulge in a cocktail at the end of the day. After three weeks, her anxiety had significantly decreased. After five weeks, her knee pain had gone away, as well as her headaches. Her rashes significantly improved around this time as well. And within eight weeks, Heather felt confident that she would forever be able to maintain this way of eating that best supported her body. She no longer experienced sugar cravings! Heather felt grounded and in control of her life. And in fact, she told me that she felt more comfortable in her own skin than she had ever remembered.

Throughout the remainder of the book, I will walk you through learning all you need to know about processed sugar: how to identify it, what to swap it out for, how to stop those sugar cravings, how to detox from the inflammation as well as elegant thinking to create subtle shifts within your thoughts in order to obtain big shifts in the way you eat. In addition, we will cover food swaps for all of the top six inflammatory foods via grocery store and recipe swaps (there are over 40 recipes in the back of this book that are free of the top six inflammatory foods). Last but not least, I will send you off with a 14-day challenge to remove processed sugar from your diet and swap it out with non-inflammatory sugar.

Join me as we forge new paths toward health and vibrancy. And remember, the perfect time to start sometimes never arrives. All you have is now. This very second could be the moment you make the decision to catapult your life forward in unimaginably beautiful ways.

Chapter 4

Panic-Stricken over Sugar

"Life begins at the end of your comfort zone."
Neale Donald Walsch

How Sugar Has a Hold on Our Psyche and What to Do About It

oes the thought of removing processed sugar from your diet panic you? If it does, you're not alone. Sugar is most people's go-to when they are stressed, tired, or hungry. Sugar gives us immediate comfort and soothes emotional distress, at least temporarily. Once, I was teaching a workshop, and at the end of the class I challenged each person to remove processed sugar from their diet for one week. This required reading labels (more to come on that in Chapter 6) and eliminating the obvious sugars like donuts, cookies, and sodas. The fear of eliminating all of these foods was nearly debilitating for Jan, one of the participants. And, she's not alone. Our society is tired, stressed and hungry. Sugar gives so many of us a place to numb that stress.

Luckily, relief came to this participant when I pulled out one of my favorite treats, Zesty Lemon Bars (recipe found in the second half of this book). Each participant took a bite and suddenly the fear melted away. Jan told me, "As long as I can eat these, I will be okay." This is when the food swap idea came to life. It is so important that we fuel our bodies *and* allow ourselves to eat tasty foods. Deprivation always ends in failure. When we deprive ourselves of calories or flavors that we love, it is incredibly challenging to maintain healthy eating as a lifelong habit.

When we first think of taking processed sugar out of our life, it can feel like life has a hold on us, rather than us having a hold on life. Truly. That may sound like an exaggeration, but I remember when I first began this journey. I was so addicted to sugar, and not in a casual way. The chemical makeup in my body was literally putting me through withdrawals! I remember telling myself each morning, "Today is the day. I will make it through the day without sugar!" Then, by 3 pm nearly every day, the craving would hit me head on. It literally felt like I had zero control over the movement of my body. Sometimes I would drive to the nearest gas station to buy a Twix bar and eat it as quickly as I could. My mantra was that if I ate it quickly enough, it didn't count. How funny is that?! The crazy part is that I had actually convinced myself to believe it.

The initial process of eliminating processed sugar from your diet can be challenging. But truth be told, if you follow my steps in Chapter 8 to stop cravings in their tracks, the physical need for processed sugar will literally drop off. It is the emotional desire for sugar that can throw you off course. For example, if you begin to look *really closely* at your thoughts, there will almost always be an event that triggers negative thinking when a craving hits. The negative thinking often creates a not so fun emotion that will increase your desire for sugar. This quickly turns into a vicious cycle.

Sugar has the ability to grab hold of us, making it incredibly challenging to kick. The number one trick that I know works when starting out on this journey is to allow yourself sweet sensations and treats, as long as they come from non-inflammatory sugars. The hardest part will be to make the *commitment* to yourself. At first, your mind will likely decide that it is scary to give up processed sugar, and that it is hard or nearly impossible. If that happens to you, I encourage you to do what has always served me well, which is to do a science experiment. Until we actually do it – remove processed sugar from our diet – we will never know if it is actually so difficult or impossible. Until we make that commitment and follow through, we have no evidence to back up our thoughts.

So, try a science experiment. Make some delicious treats from the recipes in Part 2 of this book. Stock up on fresh fruit or Medjool dates (for a caramel-like treat). Allow yourself treats when your body decides you need it, this time using ingredients that heal rather than cause dis-ease. Every single time you put those clean treats in your mouth, celebrate what you are doing. While it may seem so minor to be eating a brownie with anti-inflammatory ingredients rather than one with processed sugar – it actually is *huge!* You are creating new habits, showering your body with health and love, and all while enjoying the taste of sweetness. It is a win-win, and absolutely worthy of consciously acknowledging.

The more you acknowledge the good you are doing for yourself, the more empowered you will feel and the greater the chance that you will continue to follow through. The first two weeks are the most challenging, since, as I mentioned, it takes two weeks to remove processed sugar from your body, which means that the cravings will likely hit hard during that time and you may feel some detox (see Chapters 7 and 8 for more information on cravings and detox). The beauty is in what happens between days 10 to 14; suddenly, your body begins to shift. Your energy improves. You sleep deeply through the night. Pain begins to dissolve and digestive discomfort is magically alleviated. The number on the scale decreases, and you feel more mentally grounded and clear-headed than you have in a long time.

As one of my recent clients told me after working together for five weeks, "I feel cleaner and lighter within my *being* than ever before." This same client, the week prior, told me that she no longer had the cravings for foods with processed sugars such as alcohol, cookies, and tempting sweets. This is the power of eliminating processed sugar from your body.

The hardest part of the journey is the first few steps. My client Laura told me, "The most challenging aspect is making the commitment to change your foods. But the easiest part is to continue eating that way because of how amazing you feel." Laura came to me after experiencing six years of one major medical issue after another. During that time, she had been under anesthesia for surgery twelve times. Her life had been severely compromised by near-fatal conditions. Laura believed in healing her body with diet, yet all of her work with nutritionists and dieticians only helped her feel better in small, incremental baby steps. The knowledge she gained from them was a step in the right direction, but it wasn't enough. Laura wanted her life back. When we met, she was on disability from work because of how severely her movement had been compromised. There were very few foods she could eat without having to run to the bathroom, and she was looking to lose around 75 pounds. By following the steps laid out in this book, Laura has lost 50 pounds (and counting), she can now eat all the vegetables and fruit she wants without having to find a bathroom immediately, the pain in her body is much improved, and she is back to work and even swimming laps at her local pool. That all happened in less than a year's time. Propelling your health forward is possible, once you make the decision to try on a few new habits that give you really big returns.

While we can experience such empowerment and joy making healthy choices *that taste good*, the opposite happens when we eat processed sugar. The most common thing that triggers a craving is some sort of event. The event doesn't have to be a big, prominent event. It could be as simple as your husband looking at you funny, or your child back-talking. That event will automatically create a thought in your mind. Typically the thought shows up so fast that we don't even know it was formed, but might look something like: *If I had more energy, lost a few pounds, or were more fun, my husband wouldn't look that way at me.* The thought immediately creates an emotion, which in this example would align with defeat, depression, frustration, etc. Now, here's the direct correlation between our thoughts and the foods we eat. The moment we feel a negative emotion (also known as stress), we begin to have cravings. The cravings don't show up with slow and moderate intensity. They show up *now*, and three seconds of time seems far too long to satisfy that craving with a sweet treat. The problem is, once we eat, we quickly feel guilty for having done so. We realize that our action likely compounded the problem of not having enough energy, being unable to lose weight, or feeling less than ideal. As soon as those thoughts show up, more negative emotions and therefore, more cravings are present. Pretty soon, not only our mental and emotional stability is out of alignment, but the chemical reactions in our body from the processed sugar give us physiological cravings.

The solution is threefold. First, make sure you have anti-inflammatory treats on hand so that you swap out the unhealthy stuff for healthy foods that still taste great. Check out Part 2 of this book for tasty recipes without the inflammation. Food swapping is a crucial step that will build the foundation for your success.

Second, make sure to take note of and bask in your achievements. Emphasize the mental, emotional, and physical health you are creating for yourself when you swap out those foods. *Feel* the goodness within your body as you relish your accomplishments, big and small.

Third, when you have a negative thought – and you will – practice lengthening the amount of time between the thought and any food-related response. See if you can push past the need for a sugary comfort food or drink.

The best way I have learned to elongate the space between thought and unhealthy treat is to take seven deep breaths the second I am aware of a negative thought or craving. You can try it yourself: breathe all the way down into your belly, and then breathe out. On your outward breath, try to breathe for double the time you breathed in. For example, breathe in for three seconds and out for six seconds. Modify the time to a pace that feels good for you. This type of breath work is detoxifying, and seven breaths is just enough time to create the space you need between the thought and the reaction. Once we can see that we want the cookie/cake/soda/

wine, etc. because we are looking for comfort, we have a greater chance of reaching for our healthy food swap, which will create a positive cycle of feeling empowered. This, in turn, gives us a greater chance of repeating the new healthy habit in the near future.

An EVENT
… becomes …

A THOUGHT
… which becomes …

An EMOTION
… which turns into …

A REACTION
… and then creates …

A NEW THOUGHT
…. And the cycle continues.

Chapter 5

The Sugars That Inflame Us

"We now know that food is medicine, perhaps the most powerful drug on the planet with the power to cause or cure most disease."
Dr. Mark Hyman, M.D.

How to Swap Out the Inflammatory Sugars for Sugars That Improve Health

Sugar has such a bad rap, in general, when it comes to diet and nutrition. There are sugar detox programs, sugar avoidance counseling, and different theories that address whether or not sugar should be removed from the diet. To simplify the confusion, all of the advice I am giving you is specifically designed to remove inflammation from your body. With that said, here's what you need to know.

Not all sugar is bad. And when we begin to remove all sugar from our diet, we can feel incredibly deprived. Not to mention that you may be missing out on key nutritional components such as antioxidants, minerals, and vitamins from whole fruits.

There is often confusion about what constitutes a "no sugar" diet. Sometimes that means eating no sugar of any kind, including naturally occurring sugar. For the sake of this book and for the sake of removing inflammation from your body, it's important to remember that the sugar from whole fruit is not inflammatory. If you chose to work with an anti-inflammatory health coach, they may suggest certain types of fruits, but it all depends on your individual goal. Also important to note, eating *whole* fruit is *significantly* better for you than drinking fresh-squeezed fruit juice where the pulp and fiber has been removed, giving you a more concentrated form of sugar.

Rather than memorizing all 50+ names of processed sugar, I find it easier to focus on the types of sugars that work well for our body. There are five main non-inflammatory sugars that I use. The first is raw organic honey. It's important that it is raw, because when honey is heated up, it changes the molecular make-up and creates an inflammatory response. My second favorite sugar swap is *pure organic maple syrup*. I'm talking Vermont-style maple syrup, not Aunt Jemima's imitation maple syrup. Grade B is actually the best because it's the least refined version and, as a bonus, costs less. My third swap is whole fruits. If you are looking for something to eat that is super convenient, really fast, and extra tasty, then grab yourself a banana, apple, pear, some berries, or another fruit of your liking.

If you experience a major craving for sweets or want a delicious sweetener for baked goods, pick yourself up some Medjool dates. They are nature's natural form of caramel, and the best sugar swap in muffins, pies, cookies, and cakes. Unrefined coconut sugar is my fourth sugar swap. While it is a bit more processed, it doesn't typically inflame people and has a very low glycemic rating. For my last swap, I like to use liquid stevia. I prefer stevia in the liquid form because it is less refined and better for you. In fact, recent research shows that it has anti-bacterial properties – a fun fact for you! There are zero calories and zero sugar grams in it. Also, important to note, liquid stevia is very sweet in taste. So you can add just three to five drops to a cup of coffee or tea and have a nice sweet taste to replace the sugar that you might have put in your coffee before reading this book.

There's another type of sugar I'm often am asked about as a good sugar alternative: agave. Agave is another food that has a great reputation in the health industry, but it's a little bit tricky. Similar to honey – only more intense – agave is usually found in its processed version, and, like honey, has been changed molecularly to create an inflammatory response in the body. This response is not nearly as severe as those 50+ inflammatory sugars I told you about, but it's one that I recommend staying away from most of the time unless it is raw. If you can find raw agave, it's a lovely substitution for processed sugar as well. It is, however, a bit more challenging to find in any sort of commercial items or packaged foods.

Why is it so important to remove processed sugar from our diet when trying to eliminate the chronic inflammation in our body? Processed sugar is the number one most inflammatory food along with alcohol. Processed sugar has been deemed more addictive than cocaine itself through brain scans conducted by Dr. Lustig, endocrinologist. Processed sugar has been directly correlated to a host of conditions and dis-eases such as cancer, autoimmune disorders, thyroid and hormone dysfunction, skin conditions, depression, anxiety, obesity, lower metabolism, heart dis-ease, leaky gut, truly the list goes on and on. Remember that inflammation can show up differently in each person, because it targets the areas where you're most susceptible. So sugar will also affect each person differently. It will target those weaker, more susceptible areas in your body and will make underlying conditions more pronounced. It is truly your body's way of speaking to you.

When your knees hurt, when a rash breaks out, when your stomach is upset, when you have a chronic pounding headache, when your hormones are out of whack, or when you're feeling depressed, your body might be telling you that whatever you're giving it is not the right recipe for what it needs to succeed and to thrive. You are meant feel your very best, not in another lifetime, but right here, right now. I'm here to help that become your reality.

So let's talk a little bit about the idea of removing processed sugar from your body and from your diet. My guess is that if you've never done this before, there is a certain amount of anxiety that immediately tugs at your heart and stomach. Many times when I've conducted workshops and challenged people for the week to swap out processed sugar, there is an immediate sense of panic that overcomes each participant. True to how I live life, I always bring some sort of clean treat from one of the many recipes in the back of this book. What I hear time and time again is, "Oh, my gosh, I had no idea clean eating could taste so good!"

Some processed sugar is easy to spot: cupcakes, cookies, cinnamon rolls, alcohol. These are foods that you know even without reading the ingredients are going to have processed sugar in them – unless, of course, you're making a special food swap using non-inflammatory sugars.

As a renegade researcher, your goal is to begin reading the ingredients label. Not the nutritional fact label where it tells you how many grams of sugar or grams of carbs or grams of protein are in the product, but rather the type of ingredient that's in the product. The reason we focus on this is because you could eat a banana, which has naturally occurring fruit and lots of fiber, and it could have 15 grams of sugar in it. Likewise, you could pick up a granola bar that has 15 grams of sugar, but that sugar comes directly from cane sugar, high-fructose corn syrup, or one of the top inflammatory sugars. One food, the banana, is going to give you health. The other food, the granola bar, will degenerate the cells in your body and will cause high levels of inflammation.

My challenge to you: begin swapping out processed sugars right away – even starting today. Read every single ingredients label of every single food that goes into your mouth, because education is power. And you are here to become empowered, to gain health, to alleviate all of those chronic symptoms that have been bugging you for months or years, so that you can feel and live the life you're meant to live of health, of vibrant energy, and of joy.

If you read the ingredients on Earth's Best Apple Granola bars, you will find over three different names of inflammatory sugars. In this particular flavor, you have organic cane syrup, organic rice syrup, and organic apple juice concentrate. Of course there are additional inflammatory ingredients in this list, but based on this process of swapping out processed sugar, you would not eat this bar and therefore would avoid the additional top inflammatory ingredients, including a number of wheats, organic butter flavor, canola oil, and multiple preservatives. Instead, you could swap this out for an Apple Pie Lara Bar, a Cinnamon Apple RX bar or the classic granola bars in Part 2 of this book.

I call these types of granola bars organic junk food. And the food industry tricks us constantly with their labeling and with their marketing to make us believe that we're putting health into our bodies, when instead (while there may be some healthy ingredients), inflammatory foods that are added always counteract the clean, healthy ingredients.

So as you move on from this chapter, it is important that you know that you are not eliminating all sugar from your diet. And that you can have your cake and eat it too, quite literally. What is important is that you give yourself foods with sugars in them that do not cause an inflammatory response. Give yourself abundance rather than deprivation. As you move forward, tell yourself that you can have anything you want. You can make cookies and treats and snacks. You name it, it can either be made or found using non-inflammatory ingredients. It is this shift or this food swap that will bring you into a level of health you may have never before experienced. More importantly, these food swaps and thinking thoughts of abundance rather than depletion will allow you to continue eating this way for a lifetime. Our goal is to avoid diet mentality. This is not a, "When I lose 10 pounds, I'll go back to eating the same way" program. Because when you lose 10 pounds and go back to eating the same way, you'll just gain another 10 pounds, and the chronic inflammation will continue to show up in an array of different symptoms.

This is not a calories in, calories out type of diet either. Always remember, it's what you're putting into your body that matters so much more than *how much* you put into your body. If you are hungry, fuel yourself, and if you are full, allow your body the time and space to digest what you ate.

Chapter 6

Everything in Moderation

"Our greatest glory is not in never failing, but in rising up every time we fail."
Ralph Waldo Emerson

It's All About Perspective

It is our society's general belief that everything can be good for us in moderation. I believe in everything in moderation, at least when it comes to foods that give us health. For example, I will eat non-inflammatory sugars such as pure maple syrup or raw honey in moderation. I don't eat large amounts of it, but I have it for special occasions, or sweet treats. This is what I believe the original statement of, "Everything in moderation," came from: eating a variety of whole, natural foods that we were meant to eat.

The problem is that our societal beliefs around moderation in diet have been molded via the food industry. A number of years ago, the FDA came out with a statement saying that processed sugar should be deemed a toxin, and would be illegal if it had come onto the market as a new product. However, sugar is a multi-billion-dollar food industry. The big sugar corporations fought this statement and still do, continuing to push processed sugar into nearly every box, bag, can, and package sold in grocery stores. Sugar is hidden in everything, and because of this, we continue to eat more and more of it. The more sugar we eat "in moderation," the sicker our country continues to get.

Once, I was as deluded about this as anybody. I looked around at people who ate sugar on a daily basis, even if only the stuff that was hidden in processed foods, and felt that if they could be healthy eating those foods, then this whole sugar hype must have been blown way out of proportion. There were so many people eating processed sugar each day who appeared healthy, so sugar must not be the culprit – or so I thought.

I believed it was a narrow population that was negatively impacted by processed sugar. But the years I've been coaching have dispelled that myth. As soon as I tell people that I am an anti-inflammatory health coach, they immediately start telling me about the ailments affecting them. I kid you not: 99 percent of the people who I randomly introduce myself to as an anti-inflammatory health coach tell me about the chronic symptoms they experience, and those symptoms all have inflammation at their root. These are not just my clients, but random people I meet at the grocery store, in the post office, or at social engagements. Many of these people *appear* to be healthy on the outside, but it is the chronic toll of symptoms showing up on the inside that is so insidious. The truth is, those people who ate sugar and were *never affected by it* was in actuality a story I told myself. Most, if not all, of those people were struggling with their own symptoms, yet I had created a story convincing myself that nothing was wrong with their body.

This is natural. As humans, we judge and create stories. In fact, it is so prevalent that a large portion of my work is dedicated to helping people experience the connection between food and the symptoms that they experience, so they can get out of the stories and align with *truth*.

Going back to the statement that everything is okay for you in moderation, I have a quick question to ask you, and I'm looking for your first gut answer. *When you think of the word toxin, what comes to your mind?* For me, what comes up first are items such as bleach, household cleaning products, gasoline, or nail polish. Now, would you put a *half of a teaspoon* of bleach in your coffee each morning? Just in moderation? I'm quite certain your answer is no. Then why do we as a society believe that it's okay to eat processed sugar, which was identified as a toxin by the FDA, in moderation?

The reality is that the processed sugar we consume each day is scientifically shown to cause inflammation. Period. It is not a theory, or an idea formed by a bunch of hippies. It is truth, it is science. Because most people consume significant quantities, the inflammation becomes more than your body can handle and stacks up over time. As you can see by the timeline in Chapter 3, there have been incremental amounts of processed sugar throughout history causing health issues, yet we continue to put it into our body. It's not for a lack of knowledge (for most people), but rather processed sugar is so dang addictive, tasty, and convenient.

If you are just beginning to eat an anti-inflammatory diet and are experimenting with swapping out processed sugar, remind yourself that you are on a journey. No one is perfect. If you have fallen off the bandwagon and are trying to get back on, remember we all "fail" at times. The truth is, there is no such thing as failure, as long as you learn from your experience. In fact, I secretly get really excited when a client falls off the bandwagon, as they then have the gift of experiencing the contrast of feeling great and then not so. The "feeling bad" after eating processed sugar (or a food that does not serve your body) is simply your body speaking to you, asking you not to eat or drink that again. It's a beautiful opportunity to learn about you, and what makes you feel good. If you choose to consciously look at your experience through this lens, you will gain so much.

The idea is to keep walking toward an objective of eliminating processed sugar from your diet while eating the sugars that do not inflame you. The ultimate goal is to eat only those foods that support you rather than cause degeneration. With that said, we are human and perfectly imperfect. With each forward step you take, remember to celebrate all accomplishments, big and small. If you fall off the wagon and eat a piece of cake, the power is in hopping right back on the clean-eating train. Drink your water, eat some clean protein, and prepare your food ahead of time so success is more likely in the week ahead of you. (Look for more tips to hop back on the clean-eating train, to detox, and how to stop cravings in their tracks in the next chapter.)

When looking to eliminate inflammation from your body, the ultimate goal is to remove all processed sugar rather than to eat it in moderation. But notice, I said *ultimate.* There are two subtle ways of thinking that end in radically different scenarios. If we believe that the ultimate goal is to eat everything in moderation, and if you already have chronic inflammation stacking up in your body, then processed sugar, in moderation, could be the culprit not allowing your body to heal completely. On the other hand, if you believe that the ultimate goal *is* to swap out all processed sugar, but you are human so fall off the wagon from time to time, yet continue to take strides forward, the healing in your body will become inevitable and the inflammation will eventually fall off of you. Ultimately, an improvement is improvement, and that is what we continue to strive for. As quoted by Naeem Callaway, "Sometimes the smallest step in the right direction ends up being the biggest step of your life. Tiptoe if you must, but take the step."

Everyone has a different journey, and everyone has a different process when it comes to clean eating. With that said, clients often share in their first session with me that they eat really well, so are confused as to why they do not feel better. They typically say something like this:

"I eat a mostly healthy diet. It's pretty clean, and I exercise and take good care of myself. I can't understand why my arthritis won't go away, or why my digestive issues are so insistent. I have headaches a couple of times each week, and I feel like I'm depressed. I have really low energy. I know this is coming from inflammation, but I really do eat so well."

The truth is that the food industry and society have created a norm for eating *healthy* that in reality often creates chronic inflammation. Again, it is all perspective. When we can see the *truth* of how our body responds to the foods and drinks we consume, then we are no longer vulnerable to what others say or how great the latest food marketing scheme seems. You can't fight reality. Actually, you can, but trust me ... it traps you in that never-ending vicious cycle until you are ready to own up to your *truth.*

Sarah came to me suffering from debilitating chronic symptoms that were hampering her on a daily basis. She was a mom of two young children, owned her own business, and had an amazing life to live. The problem was that she was so sick, she could no longer live that life. Sarah would go to bed at 4:30 in the afternoon, unable to spend time after school with her children. She had to cut her work hours down to seven hours per week. She could not commit to social engagements with her friends, as she did not know if she would be in bed or able to attend the event. She longed to be able to pick up the athletic endeavors that had brought her much joy, but she was too ill. Sarah felt hopeless. She had tried the paleo diet, been to every doctor in the region, and was seeking out-of-town specialists when we began working together.

As Sarah became a renegade researcher, she followed this process and *truly listened to her body.* Sarah was able to learn what caused inflammation by *feeling* and *listening* to her body every time she ate and drank. Within six weeks of swapping out inflammatory foods for those that do not inflame, Sarah was swimming laps at the pool, reading to her kids at night, and following her dreams of becoming a successful entrepreneur. It was amazing to see how Sarah's inflammation had been impacting her relationships, her career, and her ability to have fun exercising. She got her life back. You can do that, too.

Chapter 7

Feel the Detox

"Love me like the moon intended. All the way through the darkness."
A. J. Lawless

How to Detox and Stop Cravings in Their Tracks

By this time, I think you're beginning to understand the potency processed sugar has in the body. Interestingly enough, it affects more than our physical symptoms. In fact, processed sugar has been proven, through thermal brain scans, to be as addictive as cocaine. The addiction is real for many reasons, and affects both physical and emotional aspects of the body. In this chapter, you're going to learn how to detox, how to embrace the detox, and what you can do to stop cravings (a common symptom of detoxing) in their tracks.

The goal of our "work together" is to get as much inflammation *out* of your body as possible. We know there is chronic inflammation already lurking in your body. We know it is in part due to your diet (or you wouldn't be reading this book). And, we know that if you keep doing what you've always done, then you will continue adding toxins to your body. This means the liver and kidneys will continue to work on overdrive. There will continue to be more toxins than your body can process, and one of two things will happen. Either you will feel more intense symptoms and your health condition will escalate, or your body will create fat pockets to store the toxins as far away from your organs as possible. Neither option is fun, but those are the processes that take place when we cannot get the inflammation out.

The goal of anti-inflammatory eating is to stop the flow of inflammation going *into* your body. Then we use techniques like drinking water, moving your body, Epson salt baths, deep breathing, or meditation and mindfulness to help eliminate any chronic inflammation stuck inside. This is where the detox process truly begins.

What does detox really look like and why does it happen? Detox happens when your kidneys, liver, and lymphatic system are pushing out toxins in an effort to eliminate them from your body. The detox process requires your body to once again process the inflammation to eliminate it once and for all. The effort of pushing out the inflammation can cause an array of symptoms such as headaches, nausea, irritability, tiredness, constipation, diarrhea, brain fog, sleep irregularity, bad breath, achy or flu- or cold-like symptoms, hunger, itchy skin, intense cravings, or bad body odor. Surprisingly enough, this list of symptoms is not complete when it comes to detoxing. If you have a susceptible condition, it may rear its ugly head for a couple of days during the detox before it begins to heal.

I once had a client, Sam, who had gout. While the gout did not affect him on a day-to-day basis, it was debilitating when it showed up. As Sam began to eliminate inflammatory foods and swap them out for foods that healed, his gout showed up with a strong vengeance. He was bedridden for two days as his body processed the toxins, but once the major detox was over, the pain went away as well as his gout. He no longer needed medication for gout. While the two days of detox were certainly not the highlight of his life, it was absolutely worth the freedom he experienced as the gout was eliminated from his life.

Often, when people begin to experience detox, it scares them. They may all of a sudden say, "Wait a second. I'm trying to feel better, and I'm actually feeling worse. This isn't working." Or, "I know detox is coming, but this feels so crappy I don't want to continue." I want to give you some really good news. The most intense part of detox typically lasts three to five days and it means you are on the *brink* of healing and regeneration. Remember, magic begins at the end of your comfort zone.

Detox doesn't last forever, and it's so important to embrace it in order to push through. I love to pivot my thinking during times of detox from, "This is no fun and I hate detoxing," to, "Oh, my word, I've got one raging headache! I'm so tired. And… I'm actually happy about it because I know this means the inflammation is leaving my body." When you are feeling these detox symptoms, you can be assured that the inflammation is getting pushed out of your body. This is awesome, as long you know to think about it in a way that keeps you on the clean-eating train.

Stop Cravings in Their Tracks

In addition to the physical symptoms that one may experience when detoxing, there are the food cravings. A chemical and physiological reaction is taking place in your body during this detox time that makes you crave foods, typically those that aren't good for you. I always know I'm detoxing when, all of a sudden, I want some sort of sugary treat or I want a glass of wine, which is so not how I typically eat. Yet, all of a sudden the craving is real and straight in my face.

At this point in my life, I'm grateful to be able to notice and observe my cravings, rather than react to them. That takes a lot of practice and often a bit of coaching. So, as you begin this process, I'm going to give you the top three ways that you can stop cravings in their tracks: drink water, eat clean protein, and allow yourself a sweet treat using non-inflammatory sugar.

At the first onset of cravings, the first thing you want to do is drink a large glass of water. Don't sip on it. Again, throw it back and chug it. Water actually stabilizes your blood sugar levels, lubricates your joints, supports healthy hormone production, and, of course, helps get toxins moving out of the body as quickly as possible. Interestingly enough, I find that when I'm dehydrated, those cravings become stronger. So keep a large bottle of water alongside you and remember to drink, drink, drink it. That bottle of water does you no good if it sits beside you all day, untouched.

Step two is to eat a clean source of protein. After you have drunk a large glass of water (or two), the next thing I want to make sure you do is eat a minimum of 15 grams of clean protein. We're going to talk more about what constitutes clean protein in the next chapter. This too helps stabilize your blood sugar levels and gives you a sense of grounded-ness. In addition, it supports healthy function of your immune system, fuels your muscles, and boosts your metabolism.

Ultimately, we want to attack the craving by stabilizing your blood sugar levels. Stabilizing your insulin levels supports the balancing of all of our other hormones that may have started to go off-kilter. Many people do not realize this, but the removal of inflammatory foods along with controlling insulin levels has the ability to heal hormone dysfunction. I know this personally, as I was able to get off of Armor Thyroid (a pharmaceutical thyroid medicine) after being on it for six years by following the steps outlined in this book, plus balancing my macronutrients. Eating enough clean protein every two to three hours is a major component to begin balancing your macronutrients (protein, carbs, and fat).

The third and last step to stop cravings in their tracks is to give yourself some sort of clean, sweet treat. Remember, this way of eating is not about deprivation. This is not about telling your body you can never have anything that tastes sweet again. This is about giving your body nutrients. It's about fueling your body with sweet-tasting foods that help you regenerate, rather than degenerate, on a cellular level.

So, what does that clean, sweet treat look like? It could be as simple as a pint of berries, a banana, an organic apple, or some sliced up pineapple.

It could be one of the delicious, clean, sweet treats that you'll find in Part 2 of this book. Treats like Carr Family Brownies, Ginger-Molasses Cookies, Zesty Lemon Bars, and Vanilla Chocolate Kisses. It's all possible by swapping out inflammatory ingredients for those that do not cause inflammation. It's absolutely my recommendation to make a triple batch of the recipe that you enjoy eating. This way the treats are available to you when you have a craving, *right now*. If you have to make the treats, or run to the store, more than likely you will end up reaching for something that makes you fall off the wagon.

To recap, we have talked about embracing the detox symptoms, as well as three action steps to stop cravings in their tracks. Number one, chug water. Number two, eat around 15 grams of protein. Number three, give yourself some sort of clean treat. This is absolutely huge. I have seen people who were lifetime soda drinkers quit drinking soda using these steps. People who are committed sugar-holics, whose diet was 99% sugar, eliminate and stop the cravings completely, by following these steps. These steps are transformational, so be sure that you *take action*, rather than resting in assurance that you know what to do. Knowledge is only part of the piece to solving your issues. *You must take action, as it is in the gap between knowledge and action where so many people fall down.*

5 Detox Recovery Tips

Following these next tips will push the toxins out of your body more quickly so you can experience symptoms for shorter periods of time. The first thing you can do is take an Epsom salt, or Dead Sea salt bath. Get the bath as hot as you possibly can (without burning you) and add Epsom salt (following the directions on container). Sit in that bath as long as you can, allowing yourself to sweat significantly. Sweating is one of the top two methods that you push toxins (and fat) out of your body. The second method is through elimination via urination. There are other ways to push out the inflammation, but those are the top two most effective modalities. While sweating all day may not be a reality, peeing is, which brings me to detox recovery tip number two: drinking lots of water. (Do you see a theme with the importance of water?)

You have already learned the benefit of drinking one gallon of water each day, however never is there a more important time to do so than during detox. In fact, if you don't drink enough water while your body is trying to push toxins out, it can actually reabsorb the toxins. *Drinking enough water cannot be emphasized enough.*

A third method for helping to push toxins out of your body more effectively during the detox process is to incorporate gentle movement in your daily routine. I'm not talking long runs, heavy lifting, or high-cardio workouts. The idea is to get your blood flowing, which will help pick up the toxins and inflammation so they can be more easily excreted. Movement such as light stretches, a gentle walk, bouncing on a trampoline, or playing with your child at the park are perfect ways to accomplish this recovery tip.

The fourth tip is often the most overlooked: *rest*. Rest is one of the lifestyle objectives most important for weight loss and the regeneration of health. It is especially important during detox, as your liver and kidneys are working overtime. Similar to someone who runs a marathon, these organs are exhausted during detox. To ask them to run a marathon after a night of no sleep would be nearly impossible. Rest is a tricky aspect, as sleep can be compromised for a few days at the height of detox. If you are having difficulty experiencing deep sleep, remember that rest counts when your feet are up off the floor and your eyes are closed. Your goal during detox is to carve out as much rest time in your day as possible and to begin listening to your body. If it says it's tired, set aside your to-do list and take a cat nap, or put up your feet for as long as you can.

The fifth method for supporting the detox process, which I highly encourage, is breath work. Deep breathing is another method to remove inflammation from your body. I really like the simple breath where you breathe in your nose for three counts and then you breathe out for six counts. It is the outward breath that is most detoxifying. Find a comfortable place to sit, with your back straight, close your eyes … and breathe. I have watched time and time again how as short as a two-minute meditation or breath work session each day can transform peoples' lives.

I love to breathe in and visualize my breath going into my nose, spiraling down my spine, pooling in my heart center and then leaving my mouth as a cascading waterfall on the outward breath. As I breathe out, I push my belly button against my spine and visualize all of the air coming out of my mouth. Not only are you are receiving enormous benefit when breathing to detoxify the body, but there's been a lot of research that shows mediation to be more deeply restful than sleep itself.

Chapter 8

Clean Protein Deserves a Food Category of Its Own

"Don't judge a book by its cover."
George Eliot

Clean Protein Can Be the Difference Between Degeneration and Regeneration

In the prior chapter regarding detox, we talked about one of the major action steps to stop cravings in their tracks. This is to drink a glass of water and then to *eat some clean protein,* followed by a sweet clean treat. Clean protein truly deserves a food category of its own, and it's important to make the differentiation, as it has the potential to heal or harm you on a physical level.

Many anti-inflammatory diets recommend not eating meat at all. I understand this recommendation based on the protein that most people in our modern society eat. However, it's important to make the differentiation between modern-day meats and clean protein that we have eaten for lifetimes past. Becoming a vegetarian, vegan, or omnivore is a very personal decision. I'm not here to tell you which category to eat, as each of our bodies functions uniquely and thrives from different macronutrient ratios. This chapter is not about eating meat or not, but rather about finding the type of clean protein that best suits you.

Clean beef protein comes from a life lived off of the land, a cow that has only eaten grass or hay, ever. This is important because our food industry now feeds cows genetically modified corn and soy as a standard feed. It makes sense. Corn and soy will fatten up cattle much more quickly than having them simply graze off the land. This allows the rancher to sell the cattle more quickly and make more money in an industry that requires tremendous energy, time, and devotion to making minimal money for their effort. The problem is that corn and soy are two of the most genetically modified foods on the planet. It seems that our food industry often comes down to the bottom dollar. Because genetically modified corn and soy have a higher yield, farmers can sell it to the ranchers for a much cheaper price.

In the following chapters, we will talk more in depth about why genetically modified foods are included as one of the top six inflammatory foods. What's important to know now is that genetically modified foods are directly linked to leaky gut, which appears in almost all people who have an autoimmune condition. Leaky gut often creates food allergies and ultimately creates a toxic overload systemically, as food is pushed through the intestinal lining and into the rest of the body.

When a cow eats genetically modified food, the toxins and inflammation from the GMO feed enters the body and is typically stored in the animal's fat. When we eat the beef from this cow, we're eating the toxins and inflammation that were stored in the fat and tissues of the cow. This enters our body directly and causes the same havoc in us.

It's important to note that regular, grass-fed beef is not always what it appears. True to the food industry's tricks and misleading ways, it is legal to label beef that has been *mostly* grass fed but then finished on grain as "grass-fed" beef. It's best to look for the label "grass-fed, grass-finished" on beef to ensure you are getting the clean meat you are looking for.

Moving onto poultry, the keywords you want to look for are free range, organic chicken or turkey. The free range refers to a bird that has been allowed to roam around the fields eating grass and bugs that are chalk full of omega-3 fats. The grass that cows eat and the grubs that poultry eat are full of omega-3 fats. Omega-3 fats fight off inflammation in the body. In fact, omega-3 fats are one of the greatest forms of super foods available to humans. They help to prevent Alzheimer's and dementia. Omega-3 fats help you lose unwanted fat, stabilize hormones, and help with the absorption of nutrients through your cell walls.

Fish also requires the art of detection in order to know if it's clean or not. As most of you know, fish, such as salmon, are great sources of omega-3 fats as well. However, that has begun to change in recent times as fish farms often feed fish GMO foods. In addition, fish farms typically do not have adequate space per fish, so they end up swimming around in one another's waste. When purchasing fish, remember to look for *wild* caught in order to eliminate any inflammatory components within the fish.

Eggs follow the same concept as poultry. Free range eggs are full of omega-3, inflammation-fighting fats, while traditional eggs are chockfull of GMO-formed fats that cause inflammation. There has much debate throughout the years over whether eggs are good or bad for us. The debate has mostly revolved around whether eggs create bad cholesterol in the body. What I find time and time again is that when my clients work on removing inflammation from their body (this includes eating an ample supply of omega-3 fats), the bad cholesterol rapidly declines. Again, it is not the egg that is good or bad for you, but the type of egg that determines your outcome. Please note, cage free is not the same as free range. Cage free means it's slightly more humane, and there is less confined spaced in the pen. Free range means that the chickens have been wandering around outside, eating the grass and grubs.

Why are we talking so much about protein? A lot of people don't get enough protein to fully support or meet their health goals. The minimum amount of protein that best addresses most people's general needs is approximately 100 grams of protein per day; that's approximately 20 grams of protein every two to three hours. Many people eat significantly less. This protein will help stabilize your hormones. It will support the elimination of cravings. It will fill you up and fuel your muscles. Protein supports your immune system and helps you feel more grounded. However, none of this protein does the body good unless it comes from a clean source, so take a little time, speak with your butcher, find your local ranchers, and go to your local farmers' market, where you can source these clean types of protein.

If you are vegetarian, I want to give you a few of the most highly dense vegetarian options for getting protein in your body each day. I recommend eating eggs in the morning as a great source of protein and healthy fat. Each egg is equal to approximately 6 grams of protein. I also love a high-quality protein powder (be sure to read the ingredients so it is free of the top inflammatory foods). Smoothies are an excellent way to use protein powder. Traditionally, one scoop of protein powder is equal to 15-20 grams of protein. Pumpkin and hemp seeds are exceptionally packed with protein. In one quarter cup of these seeds, there are approximately 12 grams of protein. Hemp seeds are *also* chockfull of the beloved omega-3 fats. Sprinkle them on a salad, pour them into a smoothie, add them to granola, pancakes, and bread. Additionally, legumes can be exceptionally high in protein, depending on the variety.

Nut-Busting Myths

Contrary to popular beliefs, nuts are not a great protein source. They are a fat source and typically allow you only a couple of grams of protein per serving. The same is true of dairy. While there is protein in it, the primary macronutrient is fat. So if you are eating nuts throughout the day thinking you are getting your protein in, likely you will want to swap those nuts out for a different source referenced here.

A Day in the Life of Protein – Omnivore

In order to envision what 100 grams of protein per day would look like, check this out. Start your day off with two eggs, (approximately 12 grams of protein). Two hours later, make yourself a smoothie with a scoop of protein powder for 20 grams of protein. At lunch time, you might have a salad with approximately four ounces of clean meat, maybe some salmon or turkey or thin strips of beef, and add a quarter cup of pumpkin seeds. This will give you approximately 40 grams of protein at lunch. As a mid-afternoon snack, you might have a quarter cup of hemp seeds (about 12 grams of protein), and for dinner, you could go for three to five ounces of clean meat or fish with some brown rice and roasted veggies (giving you an additional 35 grams of protein). This type of eating throughout the day will give you about 120 grams of protein per day. Of course you can modify this as needed, but I wanted to demonstrate the simplicity of allowing yourself enough protein each day.

A Day in the Life of Protein – Vegetarian

In order to envision what 100 grams of protein per day would look like, check this out. Start your day off with two eggs (approximately 12 grams of protein). Two hours later, make yourself a smoothie with one-and-a-half scoops of protein powder, for approximately 30 grams of protein. At lunch time, you might have a salad with approximately two ounces of goat cheese, one cup of beans, a hard-boiled egg, and add a quarter cup of pumpkin seeds. This will give you approximately 40 grams of protein at lunch. As a mid-afternoon snack, you might have a quarter cup of hemp seeds (about 12 grams of protein), and for dinner, you could go for one serving of organic black bean spaghetti noodles with extra virgin olive oil and roasted veggies (giving you an additional 25 grams of protein). This type of eating throughout the day will give you about 120 grams of protein per day. Of course you can modify this as needed, but I wanted to demonstrate the simplicity of allowing yourself enough protein each day.

QUICK PROTEIN MATH

- Typically one cup of beans is approximately 7-11 grams of protein.
- Each ounce of meat is equal to approximately 6-8 grams of protein.
- 1 egg is equal to approximately 6 grams of protein.
- ¼ cup hemp or pumpkin seeds is equal to approximately 12 grams of protein.
- 1 scoop of protein powder is equal to approximately 15-20 grams of protein.
- 1 serving of organic black bean spaghetti pasta is equal to approximately 25 grams of protein.

*There are other sources of protein, which may not be the main macronutrient, however certainly add up over the course of the day. A few examples are: steel cut oats, long grain brown rice, quinoa, spinach, sunflower microgreens, goat cheese, and goat yogurt.

Chapter 9

Beyond Sugar

"If you're brave enough to say goodbye, life will reward you with a new hello."
Paul Coehlo

The Additional 5 (Inflammatory Foods) and How to Swap Them Out

The magic of this process is that by swapping out processed sugar, by default, you eliminate many of the remaining top five inflammatory foods: processed wheat, cow dairy, alcohol, inflammatory oils, and genetically modified foods (GMOs). Of course, there are additional inflammatory foods in our world today. Foods like sodium, preservatives, and pesticides (which as an added bonus are mostly eliminated once you swap out the top six inflammatory foods and purchase organic). Beyond these top six inflammatory foods, each person responds to unique foods in their own way. The only way to be absolutely certain what individual foods are inflaming you is to hire an anti-inflammatory health coach or to eliminate the top six and week by week and test out the foods that are suspicious. By eliminating the foods that inflame us, we allow the body to be in an environment that supports healing. As an added bonus, removing these top inflammatory foods often causes random food sensitivities and allergies to dissipate.

Approximately every 120 days (give or take some depending on the location in the body), new cells are made through a duplication process in the spleen. My goal for you is to get the best bang for your buck when it comes to swapping out foods that will make the biggest impact on the inflammation within your body. Replacing processed sugar does just that. If you want to take it a step further, purchase organic foods as much as possible and work at swapping out these remaining top five inflammatory foods.

Once you have become a master at eliminating processed sugar from your diet, it may be fun to play around with the following foods as you swap them out, then *listen to how your body responds.* NOTE: I recommend swapping one food out at a time, for at least two weeks, being sure not to eat anything else that you know is inflaming you (like the top six inflammatory foods). Notice if you feel better. Once a food has been out of your diet for one to two weeks and you add it back in, again, *listen to how your body responds.* Do any of those chronic symptoms show up? Do you feel funky in any way? If so, my recommendation is to keep it out of your diet for as long as possible, as my experience and observation is that each of these foods significantly inflames people.

Modern-Day Wheat

Wheat is not what it used to be when our grandparents or great grandparents baked with it. Unfortunately, modern-day wheat is a totally different food than that of 50+ years ago. This is largely due to the genetically modified wheat that has overrun our country and parts of the world. The genetically modified wheat has been turned into a franken-wheat, making many people sick and extra-sensitive to gluten due to the super injected gluten in each seed.

Beyond the added gluten to modernized wheat, there is also glyphosate, the active ingredient in Roundup, found in most GMO seeds. It also causes inflammation due to the high levels of processing used when including wheat as an ingredient in packaged food. In fact, there is an active lawsuit against Roundup for the source of certain types of Lymphoma cancer.

The story of a "Wheaties" – type cereal will shed some light on how wheat has turned from food to a food-like product. Once upon time, hunters and gatherers learned how to grow crops, which helped them settle in one location to create their own civilizations. During this time, people would plough the land though animal and man power. There were no tractors driving over the earth back then or fertilizers being added to the ground.

People would plant wheat seeds that had been plucked from their neighbor's field. There was not any Roundup embedded within the seed to ensure its ability to grow and beat the chances of insect kill. There were also no hybridized seeds injected with extra gluten. The likelihood of this seed surviving was purely up to nature. If the wheat plant made it to maturity, someone would harvest the plant. The wheat was then brought to someone who specialized in grinding the wheat using a bowl and tool made out of stone. This was extra tricky because unlike modernized wheat which has been pumped full of gluten making the wheat itself quite fluffy, ancient wheat was small and coarse. The wheat would get mashed up between two stone objects until it turned into a wheat meal of sorts. (Kind of like almond meal.) This is what our ancient relatives used to cook bread with. The bread was not light and fluffy. In fact, it was thick and dense – much like what you find when you purchase Ezekiel, non-GMO, sprouted wheat bread.

Today, the Wheatie (or insert any modernized wheat product) that so many of us use and know well is made from a wheat that doesn't deserve to be classified in the same category as ancient wheat. Once the Roundup-laden seed is planted into the already chemical-soaked soil, it sprouts and matures (consistently). Due to the GMO process, this wheat is super-charged with extra gluten, ensuring our breads, cereals, and pastries have an extra-fluffy consistency to them. In turn, the extra gluten in each wheat plant over-exposes us to gluten, causing a host of inflammatory conditions. Once harvested, the chemically and genetically altered wheat is taken to a "facility" where it is heated up, chopped up and spit out as a plant our body no longer recognizes as food

Modern-day wheat is found in a host of random food-like products. It can be found hidden in everything from soups, to vodka, to lipstick, to envelope adhesive. Modern-day wheat, along with cane sugar, soy, and corn, is among the top genetically modified foods on this planet. We're going to talk more about genetically modified foods in the next section, but it's important to note there are multiple reasons that wheat causes inflammation for people.

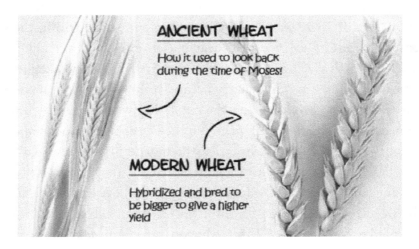

Wheat Food Swaps

Everyone has their unique make-up as to what their body can tolerate, however I have found that small amounts of an ancient sprouted wheat in a bread that uses no processed sugars, or cow dairy, or other inflammatory oils works well for most people. Of course, the key is listening to your body to see if symptoms arise after eating the ancient sprouted wheat.

Note: If you have an autoimmune condition, it is probably best to stay away from wheat altogether until your body heals. One of the food swaps I love to give my kids to replace modern-day wheat bread is Ezekiel Bread. Ezekiel Bread is a more dense bread (much less gluten), and is made from sprouted grains, which means it is less processed. You can find it in the freezer section of most grocery stores. In addition to all of these benefits, Ezekiel bread is one of the few grocery store bread options without processed sugar. It tastes fabulous toasted with extra virgin coconut oil spread over the top. For a fluffy-in-texture bread, try my Fluffy Sandwich Bread when can be found at the start of the recipes section of this book. This recipe is grain-free and made in a blender! It doesn't get much easier to make bread than that.

Some additional wheat swaps are coconut paleo wraps for sandwich rolls and sprouted non-GMO corn tortillas for tortillas swaps. In Part 2 of this book, you will find recipes for pancakes, muffins, cakes, cookies, pizza, and more using coconut and almond flour as wheat flour substitutes. Last, I love to use Tinkyada organic brown rice pasta as a traditional pasta replacement. While there are a number of different gluten-free pastas out there, I find Tinkyada pasta to be the most consistent in texture and taste to traditional pasta. In fact, many of my clients swap it out at home and their families never know the difference!

Cow Dairy

Lactose is a naturally occurring sugar found in cow dairy. When found in its natural form, lactose is not the culprit that causes large amounts of inflammation in the body. However, the processed sugars such as corn syrup, cane sugar (even if it's organic – or any other inflammatory sugar) often found in flavored dairy is the sugar you want to stay away from. Beyond the sugar, cow dairy is inflammatory for even more reasons. To begin with, the protein molecule in cow dairy is quite large. It's so large that our body doesn't easily digest it.

Beginning at birth until around the age of three, our body creates extra digestive enzymes that help to break down larger protein molecules.

This bodily function is created from an evolutionary process. Going back to the cavemen days, people would breastfeed their children until around the ages of three or four. To adapt to a larger intake of milk, infants and toddlers are able to digest cow milk because their bodies have the necessary digestive enzymes. Slowly, as they mature, children become less capable of breaking down the larger sized protein molecule.

In addition to the difficulty people have digesting cow milk, it often creates inflammation because of the feed it is given, generally genetically modified corn and soy. Corn and soy are what primarily make up feed for most cows. The inflammatory properties of the GMO corn and soy enter the cow's body, including the milk. When we ingest that milk, yogurt, ice cream, or cheese, it in turn inflames us. You may wonder if grass-fed cow dairy would be a better option. My answer is, yes, however you still have to deal with the large protein molecules and yet another issue, below, that causes inflammation in the body from cow dairy.

Issue number three that causes inflammation in cow dairy are the hormones and antibiotics commonly used by dairy farmers. In order to ensure cows provide enough milk for long enough periods of time, cows are often given growth hormones and antibiotics. Similar to beef, these hormones and antibiotics are passed on to the consumers eating the dairy.

Cow Dairy Food Swaps

There are a number of cow dairy swaps that work really well. As a milk alternative, I prefer organic canned coconut milk, goat milk, or homemade nut or seed milk. The reason I recommend either canned coconut milk or homemade nut/seed milk is because many of the milk alternatives found in boxed cartons are full of inflammatory oils, preservatives, and often sugar.

When swapping out yogurt, I love either goat or sheep yogurt. Both of these yogurts will need to be purchased in their plain form, without sugar. My trick to add a bit of pizazz is to mix approximately three droppers full of vanilla crème, mixed berry, lemon, or orange-flavored liquid stevia into one serving of plain yogurt. To add even more depth of flavor, find a food-grade essential oil and add two to three drops of lemon or orange essential oil with the complementary stevia flavor. Mix in some organic frozen berries, and you have one delicious treat, packed with a substantial amount of clean protein.

Cheese is often a food people really miss when eliminating cow dairy. Luckily, in recent years an array of goat and sheep cheeses has become available. Goat cheese is no longer defined as just that stinky, soft cheese crumbled onto salads. You can now find cheddar, mozzarella, and even jack-flavored goat cheese. I specifically use the brands Alta Dena and Mt. Sterling goat cheeses to melt on quesadillas, grilled cheese sandwiches, and lasagna. Manchego sheep cheese is another favorite that can be shredded and melted for a slightly richer flavor. Note: Many of the nut and rice cheese substitutes use canola oil or other common inflammatory oils.

The last cow dairy swap that is near and dear to many peoples' hearts is ice cream! While I have only found one company that uses non-inflammatory sugars, they have many flavors and are absolutely delicious! Coconut Bliss ice cream seems to stand in integrity with their ingredients. They are also easy to find in local grocery stores. So go ahead and have a guilt-free bowl of ice cream on me.

A quick note about goat and sheep dairy, and why the body responds better to it. The smaller the animal, the smaller the protein molecule found in the dairy. This is important because we have digestive enzymes that can more easily break that protein down. In addition, because it's goat and sheep, it likely doesn't have the same antibiotics and hormones as that of cows (although that may be changing as the demand for goat and sheep dairy increases). Last, goat and sheep are traditionally set out to graze rather than fed GMO feed, again noting that this trend could potentially change with the increase of demand for goat and sheep dairy.

Alcohol

Alcohol itself is highly inflammatory. It turns into a sugar in our body and is *tied with processed sugar for the number one most inflammatory food.* Unfortunately, it can be one of the trickiest foods to swap out, as it is tied so closely with social settings and one's desire to unwind after a long day. There is of course a slew of conflicting information in regards to alcohol and whether or not it is good for you. Remember, my focus is primarily on eliminating inflammation from the body. While there are excellent health benefits, for example, that can be reaped from the antioxidants found in the grapes used to make wine, sadly the alcohol wipes out much of the good that comes from the antioxidants.

Beyond the problem of alcohol causing massive amounts of inflammation, I have a few fun facts about wine that just may make you think twice before picking up your next glass. Fifty-one percent of all US wine is actually manufactured by three giant wine conglomerates. There are 76 chemical additives approved in the US by the FDA for use in making wine, including copper, ammonia, and many more. US wines are often made with genetically modified commercial yeast. Ninety-nine percent of US vineyards are irrigated and fed synthetic fertilizers. Monsanto's Roundup is the most common herbicide used in US vineyards today. Top-selling approved additives used by the US wine industry include "mega purple," which is a coloring agent. Residual sugars, fructose and glucose, are commonly left present in wine to appeal to the US consumer's sweet palate. Sugar in wine can be as high as 300 grams per liter.

I realize wine is not the only source of alcohol, yet I find it to be the most commonly debated topic in the world of nutrition and whether or not alcohol can be good for you. There's always a way to tweak research or find the good in things, yet truth is *truth*. I challenge you to a science experiment. Eliminate alcohol completely for two weeks to see how your body responds. (*It takes approximately two weeks for the inflammation from alcohol and processed sugar to pass fully through your body.*) At two weeks, determine how you're feeling. Are your chronic symptoms reducing, or gone? If so, it's no coincidence.

Often this experiment is easier than people think. I once worked with a woman named Katie. Katie was 23 years old and lived in a ski town that knew how to party. She was single and loved to go out on the town with her friends, yet she had a deep desire to also take care of her body by following an anti-inflammatory diet. Katie decided to participate in a little two-week science experiment to see how good she felt when not consuming alcohol. After two weeks, she was convinced that she wanted to continue living this way. She felt so much more grounded and in control of her life.

In order to have fun and maintain this lifestyle while still socializing with friends, Katie discovered a trick that made it easy to be social and enjoy herself without drinking alcohol. The trick was to have some sort of fun cocktail glass filled up with sparkling water (maybe even a tiny splash of cranberry juice) and a twist of lime. The *key* was to have it in an actual cocktail glass of some sort. What she discovered was that drinking was much less about the alcohol itself, and much more about feeling a sense of belonging with a group of people. When you have a fun mock-tail in your hand, not another soul needs to know it is non-alcoholic. Even if you are not drinking for a social occasion, simply having something special like a unique and fun mock-tail to sip on at the end of the day is often just as satisfying as an alcoholic cocktail itself.

Katie was able to go out on the town and attend the vast array of social engagements with her friends without ever feeling like the odd duckling. She set an example of *living*.

Alcohol Drink Swaps

I believe there are three key components to swapping alcohol out of your diet. Number one, make a drink that you do not often have. Something that, like a glass of wine, you may traditionally only consume one time at night. An example of this is purchasing coconut water with mint sprigs and a couple of raspberries to set inside a glass. It could also be sparkling water with a splash of juice (not from concentrate) and a twist of lime. You could even muddle up some berries and mint, add it to sparkling water, and mix in a few drops of vanilla crème stevia. You get the idea. It's about having fun and being creative with a drink that you do not drink often. The second key component is adding your drink to an actual cocktail glass of some sort. For example, I like to pour organic coconut water with mint sprigs and raspberries into my great-grandma's crystal wine glass. It feels so special and celebratory! The last key component is to always have a plan or mock-tail with you when you know you will be in social settings. Similar to clean eating, when we do not have a plan or swap available to us, it is significantly more challenging to stay on the wagon.

Inflammatory Oils

Inflammatory oils are similar to processed sugar in the sense that it is easier to focus on what you can eat, rather than what does not work. Generally speaking, vegetable oils cause inflammation, as do many seed oils that are heated. Last, trans-fats are not only inflammatory, but illegal in most countries because of their extreme toxicity. Unlike common thinking, fats do not make you fat and sick. Just like *clean protein* has the ability to heal the body, so do anti-inflammatory oils such as organic, extra virgin, cold-pressed olive, coconut, and avocado oils.

Avocado and coconut oils can be heated at higher temperatures, so they are ideal for cooking. The higher the polyphenol content in olive oils, the stronger the anti-inflammatory properties they hold. When the correct oils are eaten, they support your body's ability to absorb nutrients at a cellular level, they support healthy hormone production, they can increase your metabolism, and they can help prevent Alzheimer's and dementia.

Genetically Modified Foods (GMOs)

When we eat foods, our body is designed to scan the DNA in that food to identify whether or not the food is indeed something the body welcomes, or potentially an invader. Genetically modified foods have DNA that has been altered from the original state we were intended to eat. When we consume these GMO food-like products, the body perceives a threat and that an invader is entering the body. This puts the immune system on overdrive, ultimately compromising its effectiveness. In addition, GMO foods have been directly linked to Leaky Gut Syndrome, a condition linked to most autoimmune conditions and digestive disorders.

The most common GMO foods are corn, soy, cane sugar, wheat, and canola oil. Unless labeled *certified non-GMO*, these products are almost always GMO, so be sure to look for that label.

Chapter 10

Your Why

"He who has a why can bear almost any how."
Friedrich Nietzsche

Inspiration from Within

I have always told people that we could end war if everyone adopted an anti-inflammatory diet. Of course, there is a bit of sarcasm in this statement, yet there is much truth as well. You see, when you remove these inflammatory foods, you free up the liver to do its job, which is to process toxins. Further, when our liver is constantly in overdrive pushing out too many toxins, it rarely gets to effectively focus on its secondary job of creating neurotransmitters. This means that most of us walk around feeling a bit less grounded. We may experience different levels of brain fog, and likely our hormonal and emotional state is compromised.

When I started my own journey toward eliminating inflammation, I did it to feel better physically and get my identity back. Yet, the greatest gift I received was feeling better mentally. While my identity did not change, my ability to experience joy in my "new" life (with kids) arose. In the past eight years, I have been faced with adverse and highly stressful situations. The truth is, we are all faced with high levels of stress on a daily, monthly, and yearly basis. Because I feel more grounded and level-headed, I am able to respond rather than react to stressful situations with much more ease than before changing my eating and lifestyle habits. For me, this has been the pot of gold at the end of the anti-inflammatory eating rainbow.

Beyond changing my diet, there have been some key lifestyle shifts that have greatly supported my body's ability to heal in adversity. The first, and one of the most important lifestyle habits to adopt is *deep breathing*. Do you know that the average person only uses the top third of their lung's capacity? Believe it or not, breathing deeply not only helps alleviate stress, but on a physiological level, breathing out will also push inflammation out of the body. I find that five, *or even two*, minutes of sitting quietly and breathing deeply has the potential to completely shift my day. I am ten times more effective in getting myself ready and my kids out the door if I have taken that each morning to *breathe*.

Rest is the second lifestyle shift that supports our body to heal. To be honest, I find this is one of the most challenging shifts to make, maybe even more challenging than eliminating your favorite cookie or cocktail after work. Our society has been forced into permanent overdrive. We are all striving to be the best moms and dads, the best employee or entrepreneur, the most athletic, the best friend, the best sister, daughter, cousin, or aunt. We often volunteer to help make a difference in this world, even though our to-do list never seems to get shorter. In fact, it is quite the opposite. The more we accomplish, the longer our to-do list becomes. This is why rest has become such a needed component in order to allow your body to heal. The process of pushing out toxins and inflammation requires a large amount of energy from the body. Because we have only so much energy available to us on each given day, that energy can be used to run errands, to pack our kids' lunches, to volunteer, to go for runs, or to get caught up in drama around us, or we can choose to rest and save the energy that would have been used for tasks such as those above so our bodies can heal on a cellular level.

Did you know that the liver works at its highest function around 3 am? Ensuring we get adequate amounts of sleep and rest during the night is a key function for supporting the liver so it can do its best at pushing inflammation out of your body. How many hours of sleep each person needs is somewhat individualized. As I heal from the bacterial spirochete and parasite infection, I find that my body requires an average of 10 hours of sleep each night. As you regain health, you will find that you need less sleep. Your body will move from a state of healing to a state of thriving.

Sleep isn't the only method of rest. The practice of sitting still, putting your attention on your breath, and breathing deeply has been proven to be three times more restful than sleep itself. So if you are having a difficult time sleeping (which I promise will improve soon), schedule in a little extra deep breathing time so you can support your body's healing with rest.

Last, setting up boundaries (and sticking to them) is one more crucial component that supports your body's ability to rest. This goes back to wanting to be good at everything – as a parent, friend, daughter, sister, colleague, entrepreneur, volunteer, athlete, etc. Sadly, we are not able to do it all AND get the rest necessary on this healing journey. Taking some time to identify what is most important to you and then aligning your actions (what you put effort into on a daily basis) with the desired outcome (your desire to heal a physical discomfort in the body, to feel better mentally, to lose weight, etc.) is the means to success. This requires that you set boundaries and practice saying no to things taking up that precious energy and stopping you from following through with self-care.

The last lifestyle habit that will help to propel you into health is movement. I call this movement rather than exercise because for some people, gentle movement is more deeply healing than intense exercise such as going for a run or lifting heavy weights. When it comes to movement, our needs vary greatly. What is important to remember in the goal of moving the body to support the removal of inflammation is to simply get your blood flowing. This increase in circulation will help push toxins out of your body. Simple movements such as gentle stretching, yoga, and walking are excellent methods to support your body as it heals. On the complete opposite end of the spectrum are people who already exercise intensely. Again, what each person's body requires to live vibrantly varies greatly. It is important to note that too much extreme exercise will actually cause inflammation in the body. If this intense movement is happening on rare occasions, it's not a problem; however, if you are pounding the ground or lifting heavy weights each day, the tearing of the muscle – which is responsible for rebuilding muscle – does cause inflammation. It's not a problem, as long as enough rest is incorporated into your training schedule. Hence, one more example of where rest is the key to healing your body, and in this case, to improving your athletic performance.

I invite you to try on some of these lifestyle shifts and pretend they are a science experiment. Be consistent by showing up for yourself each day for two weeks and note (in a journal) how you feel before and after adopting each of these new habits. Not only will they feel good, but they will propel you into a supercharged state of healing coupled with my steps for following an anti-inflammatory diet.

There are many reasons to postpone the actions required to begin feeling better. You can continue living your life with pain, with digestive discomfort, or maybe inflammation is showing up for you in the form of exhaustion. Ultimately, changing your diet and lifestyle is *not* about eliminating the symptoms. Yes, your body will feel better, but the *why* to making these symptoms go away goes much deeper. For example, if you have digestive disorders, does it stop you from having the social life that you want? Does the inability to lose weight compromise your confidence when trying to form new relationships? Does the pain in your body stop you from running your next 5K race or perhaps playing with your grandchildren? If it is hormonal imbalance, is that preventing you from starting the family you have dreamed of? There is a *WHY* that is underneath your discomfort, underneath the pain and ailments that you experience. The why is how those symptoms are stopping you from living the life you dream of. Find your why and write it down below. Make this be the reason you commit to yourself. It's not about losing the weight, or feeling better physically. It's about enjoying life the way you want to.

What is your *why*? What will inspire and motivate you to adopt and maintain an anti-inflammatory diet?

_____

_____

_____

_____

_____

Now, I invite you to begin this journey with your *why*. Ask for help when you need it. I am cheering you on along the way! Believe in yourself, and know that there is a stranger out there who believes in you too. You can do this. It is the small steps taken each day that lead to complete transformation. Every small step deserves a huge celebration. I will congratulate you along the way, as you step up to be the change you wish to see in our world.

Chapter 11

The Gap Between Knowledge and Action

"The distance between your dreams and reality is called action."
Unknown

I t is in the gap between knowledge and action where so many people fall down. Now that you have read this book, you *have* the knowledge. The question is, will you put it into *action?*

Before I was an anti-inflammatory health coach, I was a middle school teacher. I *loved* teaching, working with kids, and helping them improve their lives socially, emotionally, and academically. I remember going to teacher in-service days and sitting through inspiring and highly educational training. So many great ideas were shared, and I always felt a sense of excitement to implement those ideas in my classroom. However, as soon as the training was over, I would go back to my classroom, sit at my desk, and feel an incredible sense of overwhelm. There were *so many* great ideas. So much knowledge had been gained, yet I didn't know where to begin ... what to implement first. And if I did implement something, I often lacked the accountability to keep it going throughout the year – unless of course I had a coach helping me along the way to brainstorm potential obstacles and problem-solve how I would work around them (thank you Michelle Rooks)! The same is true for us all, reaching out for help whether it be to a coach, family member or friend can be the missing key to success and accountability.

Watch Out for Falling Rocks!

As you adopt anti-inflammatory eating, there will be obstacles that fall into your path. You will likely take a trip, go out to eat, attend a birthday party, celebrate a holiday, or have a girls' night out. There will be times your grandma or mother-in-law makes you cookies and tells you how much it means to her if you eat them. You will have to face moments when your husband thinks you're crazy to eat this way and others judge you for how *strict* you are. (Hint – they are simply projecting their own judgments of themselves onto you.) At times you may feel stuck, making three dinners each night, one each for your kids, your husband, and yourself.

Challenges, doubts, and falling off the wagon all come with the territory. But if you really think about it, have you ever adopted a new habit that did not come with the need for a little problem-solving? The more we are open to finding ways around these obstacles, the more successful we become in living an anti-inflammatory lifestyle, rather than experiencing a two- to six-week diet. While the two to six weeks feels amazing, if we go back to our old habits we can cause more damage by thinking thoughts like: "I'm never going to be able to get it right." "I'm such a failure." Or, "I'm just meant to be overweight and sick." The truth is that somewhere along the line, you fell off the wagon (as most of us experience at some time) and forgot to stand back up in order to continue walking forward. Falling off the wagon is not what harms us – it is the not getting back on that limits our future.

Feeling Better

One of the reasons I love anti-inflammatory eating is because you feel better really quickly. Within two weeks of becoming a renegade researcher and truly eliminating processed sugar while increasing your water intake, your life could be completely transformed. And the better we feel, the more we want to celebrate. Celebrating each small (and big) step is a crucial component of this process. However, it is important to choose celebrations that reflect healthy living rather than celebrating how good we feel with a pint of Ben and Jerry's. Ironically, the better we feel, the less motivation we sometimes have to continue eating an anti-inflammatory diet.

A past client Kristen recently shared her story with me. She had been diagnosed with cancer a number of years ago and quickly changed her diet, which she religiously maintained for a solid year. After incredible healing, Kristen began to slowly eat foods that inflamed her ... because she no longer had the motivation to eat quite as well. She was in remission and she felt *so much better.* Bit by bit, one piece of pizza at dinner turned into weekly meals. Three bites of chips at a party turned into daily road snacks. Her once-perfect score of drinking a gallon of water each day turned into a few glasses. Alcohol showed up for weekly cocktail hour, and trips to the ice cream store were too good to pass up. All of the little bites here and there became "gateway drugs" that slowly led back to old ways of eating.

Along with the old food habits came past symptoms. Kristen's energy declined significantly. Her stomach seemed constantly bloated. She tried to go back to an anti-inflammatory diet, but it felt so hard. She was caught in story, the story that eating clean was hard. The *truth* is that there is nothing easier than grabbing some fruit from the store, a few organic nuts, and some clean protein to munch on. It's less expensive and time-consuming than going out. The *truth* is that clean eating is as easy as it gets, from a logistical point of view.

Food truly has the ability to heal our body. The confusion often lies between connecting our symptoms with the foods we eat. When people go to the Mayo Clinic or other major healing centers, they are told they have an inflammation-based condition, but are not always given a name for it. They feel hopeless and are desperate to get their lives back on track. They have tried different diets to support their health, only to find it improves their symptoms minimally. Sometimes these people have been able to make large and impactful shifts in their diet, but maintaining that method of eating is unrealistic. They fall off the wagon, which triggers more inflammation in the body and exasperates the symptoms. This adds to the feeling of hopelessness. The correlation between healing and diet becomes incredibly confusing and they don't know where to turn.

Luckily, if you know there is inflammation in your body, then following my anti-inflammatory protocol will, by default, support the elimination of the inflammation hence freeing up the symptoms that suck up all of the resources available to you. The tricky aspect to following an anti-inflammatory diet is that there are no governing bodies or set regulations determining what an anti-inflammatory diet really is. If you Google anti-inflammatory diet, you will find people sharing anti-inflammatory recipes using organic cane sugar and whole wheat flour! Some people define eating an anti-inflammatory diet as simply adding many of the spices (such as Ceylon cinnamon, turmeric, black pepper, cayenne, ginger, garlic etc.) into their diet. These spices absolutely have anti-inflammatory components and are fabulous to add to your cooking. However, if you have not eliminated the top inflammatory foods and swapped them out with ingredients that allow the body to heal, you will not eliminate *the root of the problem*.

These two methods are the difference between covering up a wound with a band-aid and hoping the band-aid will stick versus allowing the wound to heal with proper cleaning and rest. One method allows you to heal and forget the wound ever existed, while the other method requires that you tend to the wound on a daily basis. I invite you to ask yourself, do you want to continue tending to your wound (or symptoms) each day? Or would you prefer to buckle down and support your body as it finds the perfect environment to heal by eliminating the inflammation in your body? If you want to truly heal, these top inflammatory foods will need to come out of your diet.

The challenge often lies in our thinking. The tricky part is to get out of the stories we tell ourselves and *listen* to how our body responds. Our body never lies.

Conclusion

There you have it: the top six inflammatory foods and what to swap them out with. Even better, you now know the streamlined approach to removing most of these top inflammatory foods by becoming a renegade researcher and swapping out processed sugar for non-inflammatory, naturally-occurring sugars. Add in a daily dose of water (shoot for 128 ounces), and you will be well on your way to eliminating massive amounts of inflammation from your body. The cells inside you will begin to regenerate as you *grow young* and most importantly, the inflammation-induced symptoms that you experience on a day to day basis will begin to melt away. Sounds good, right? As the famous healer Hippocrates once said, "Let food be thy medicine and medicine be thy food."

I believe in you. Even though we have not formally met, I know you are reading this book for a reason. By making it this far, you are already stepping up to do the work. You deserve a healthy body. You deserve to feel confident in your own skin. You deserve a life free of chronic symptoms. You deserve to live without needing to take medications. *You deserve to grow young.* And in fact, not only do you deserve these things, but your body was innately designed to live and function this way. Want to see what your body is able to accomplish? Put your body into a state of healing, and let it show you.

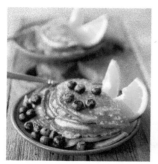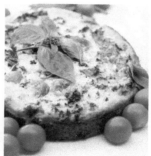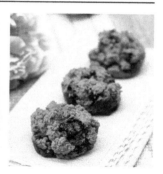

Food Swap Recipes

for Breakfast

(Be sure to check out the traditional inflammatory foods at the bottom of each recipe, so you can continue to learn what is inflammatory and how to swap those out for non-inflammatory ingredients.)

Recipes Free Of: Processed Sugar, Wheat, Cow Dairy, Inflammatory Oils & GMOs

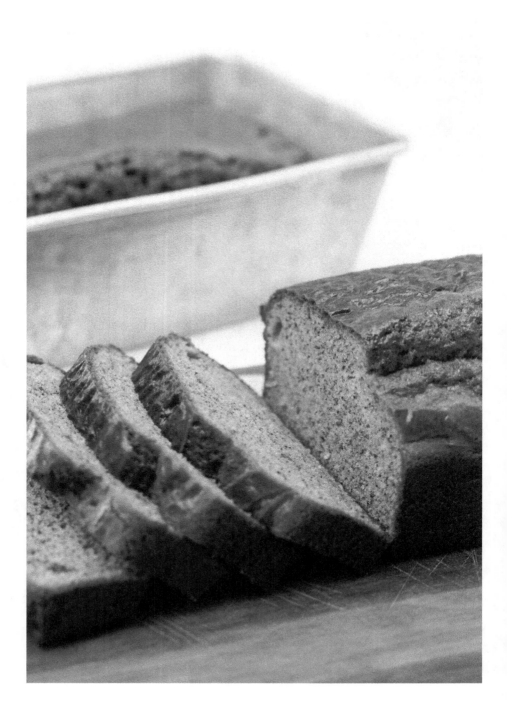

Fluffy Sandwich Bread

INGREDIENTS:
3/4 cup almond butter
6 free-range eggs
2 tablespoons raw honey
¼ cup coconut oil, melted
½ teaspoon apple cider vinegar
¼ cup ground golden flax
3 tablespoons coconut flour
1 teaspoon baking soda
½ teaspoon sea salt

INTRUCTIONS:
1. Preheat oven to 350 degrees. Line an 8 x 4"loaf pan with parchment, grease well with coconut oil.
2. In a blender, combine all ingredients and blend allowing the eggs to froth.
3. Pour mixture into greased and lined pan.
4. Bake for 35-40 minutes or until golden brown.
5. Remove from oven and allow the bread to cool in the pan 10 minutes. Remove from pan by pulling up on the parchment. Set on wire rack to cool completely.

Serves 1 loaf of bread

Standard Sandwich Bread Ingredients
(Inflammatory Foods Highlighted in Bold Italics)
Whole Wheat Flour, Water, *Sugar*, *Wheat Gluten*, Yeast, *Raisin Juice Concentrate*, *Wheat Bran*, *Molasses*, *Soybean Oil*, *Salt*, *Monoglycerides*, *Calcium Propionate*, *Calcium Sulfate*, Vinegar, *Citric Acid*, *Soy* Lecithin, *Non-fat Milk*

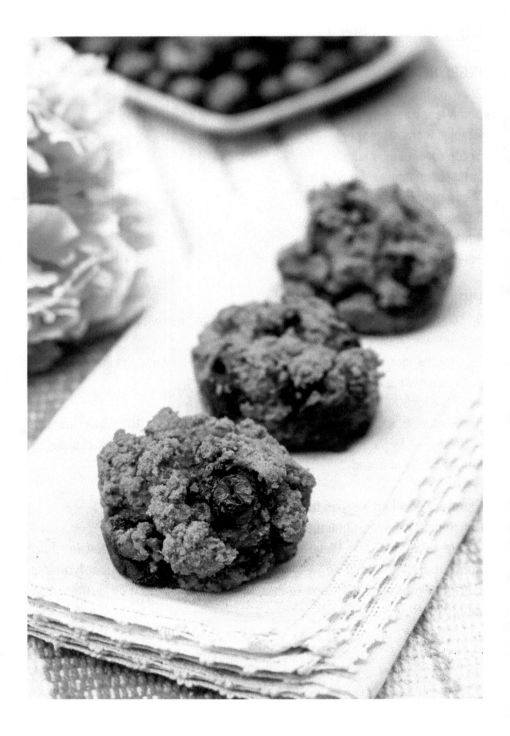

Anti-Inflammatory Blueberry Muffins

INGREDIENTS:
2 ½ cups almond flour
1 tablespoon coconut flour
¼ teaspoon sea salt
½ teaspoon baking soda
½ teaspoon pure vanilla extract
¼ cup virgin coconut oil (softened)
¼ cup pure maple syrup
¼ cup canned lite coconut milk (unsweetened)
2 free-range eggs
1 cup fresh or frozen organic blueberries
2 tablespoons ground cinnamon

INSTRUCTIONS:
1. Preheat oven to 350 degrees. Line a 12-count muffin tin with paper linings.
2. In a mixing bowl, combine almond flour, coconut flour, sea salt, and baking soda. Stir to combine.
3. Pour in coconut oil, eggs, maple syrup, coconut milk, and vanilla. Mix well.
4. Fold in blueberries and cinnamon.
5. Distribute evenly into muffin tins.
6. Sprinkle with additional cinnamon.
7. Bake for 22-25 minutes or until golden on top.

Serves 12

Standard Blueberry Muffin Ingredients
(Inflammatory Foods Highlighted in Bold Italics)
All-Purpose Flour, Light Brown Sugar, Granulated Sugar, Egg, Vanilla Extract, ***Milk,*** Blueberries, ***Salt,*** Ground Cinnamon, ***Unsalted Butter,*** Baking Powder

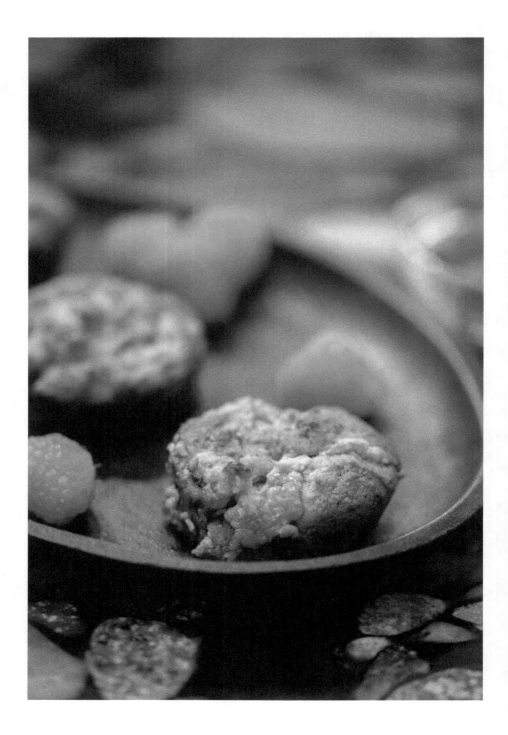

Raspberry Coconut Muffins

INGREDIENTS:
2 cups almond flour
2 whole eggs
¼ cup coconut oil, softened
¼ cup honey
1 tablespoon vanilla extract
½ teaspoon almond extract
1 teaspoon apple cider vinegar
½ teaspoon baking soda
¼ teaspoon sea salt
1 cup fresh (or thawed and strained) raspberries
12 muffin liners

INSTRUCTIONS:
1. Preheat oven to 350 degrees and line a muffin tin with 12 paper liners. (You will want muffin liners or Silpat muffin tins for these muffins.)
2. Combine all the ingredients, except for the raspberries, and mix thoroughly.
3. Gently fold the raspberries into the batter.
4. Using a ¼ cup measure, drop batter into muffin liners and bake for 15 minutes at 350F, turning the pan halfway through for even baking. The final muffins should be golden brown around the edges and firm in the center.
5. Allow to cool in the pan for 15 minutes.
Serves 12

Standard Raspberry Muffin Ingredients
(Inflammatory Foods Highlighted in Bold Italics)
All-Purpose Flour, Granulated Sugar, Egg, Vanilla Extract, Whole ***Milk,*** Blueberries, ***Salt,*** Ground Cinnamon, ***Butter,*** Baking Powder

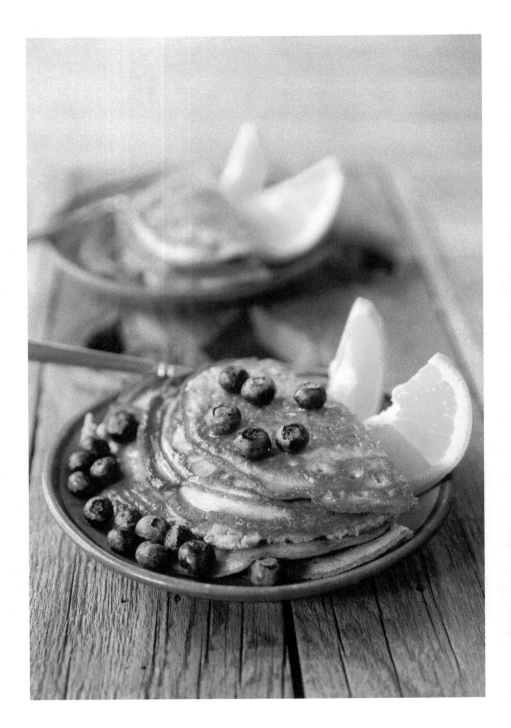

Protein Pancakes

INGREDIENTS:
10 free-range eggs.
1 ½ scoops of a clean vanilla protein powder (I recommend SunWarrior Classic, or Jay Robb protein powder - neither currently have filler ingredients such as soy, oils, sugar, etc.)
1 teaspoon vanilla extract
1 medium banana
½ orange, peeled
Coconut oil to cook the pancakes

INSTRUCTIONS:
1. Blend all ingredients together in a blender for approximately 50 seconds.
2. Cook in coconut oil.
3. Eat plain (the banana and orange gives a nice sweet taste), or top with RAW honey, berries, or pure maple syrup.

Note: These are more like crepes, which makes it easy for my toddler to eat without pieces crumbling to the ground. We so love these, and hope your family does as well!

Serves approximately 12 pancakes

Traditional Packaged Pancake Mix Ingredients
(Inflammatory Foods Highlighted in Bold Italics)
Enriched* Flour Bleached Flour, Partially Hydrogenated Soybean and/or Cottonseed Oil, Leavening, Dextrose, Salt.

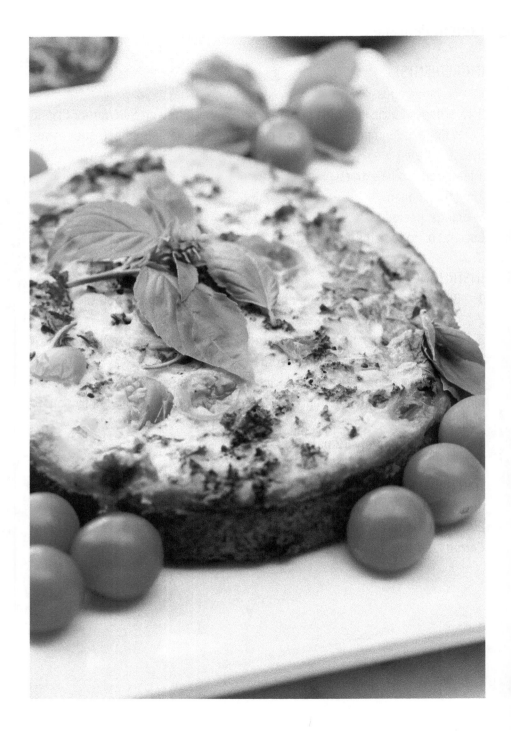

Slow Cooker Frittata

INGREDIENTS:
1 ½ tablespoons extra virgin olive oil
3/4 cup diced onion
1 ½ cups shredded goat mozzarella cheese
5 eggs
4 egg whites
3 tablespoons unsweetened coconut or almond milk
½ teaspoon ground pepper
1 ½ cups (packed) chopped baby spinach, with stems removed
1 ½ Roma tomatoes, diced
Sea salt to taste

INSTRUCTIONS:
1. In a small skillet, add coconut oil. Sauté onion on medium heat until tender, about 5 minutes.
2. Lightly grease the inside of the slow cooker with coconut oil or extra virgin olive oil.
3. In a large bowl, combine sautéed onion, 1 cup of goat mozzarella, and remaining ingredients; whisk to combine, and pour into slow cooker.
4. Sprinkle remaining cheese on top of egg mixture. Cover, and cook on LOW for 1–1 ½ hours, or until eggs are set and a knife inserted in the center comes out clean.

Serves 6

Traditional Frittata Ingredients
(Inflammatory Foods Highlighted in Bold Italics)
Eggs, *Parmesan Cheese,* Black Pepper, *Salt, Butter,* Sautéed Vegetables, *Sliced Deli Meat,* Dried Herbs

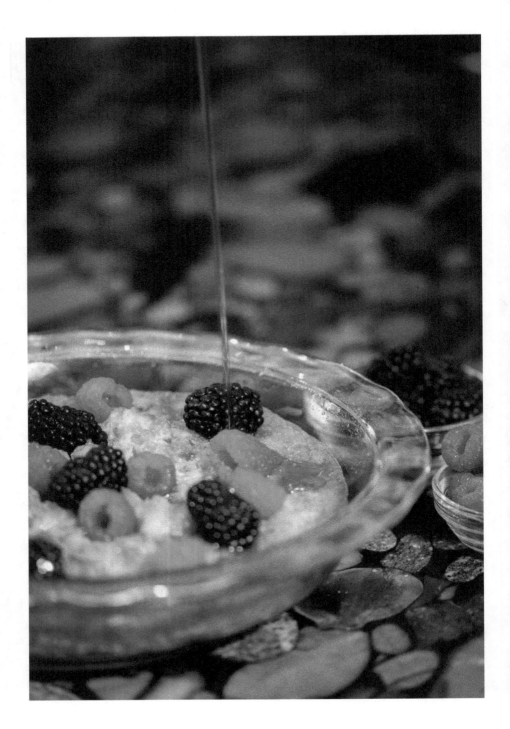

German Pancakes

INGREDIENTS:
9 free-range eggs
¼ cup extra virgin coconut oil
1 cup canned light organic coconut milk
⅓ cup coconut flour
1 tablespoon vanilla extract
¼ teaspoon sea salt
Pure organic maple syrup and berries to taste

INSTRUCTIONS:
1. Preheat oven to 425 degrees.
2. While the oven is preheating, melt coconut oil in a glass cake or pie pan in the oven.
3. Blend all ingredients together (minus the coconut oil, maple syrup, and berries) in a blender for 30-60 seconds.
4. Pour mixture into the heated pan.
5. Bake for approximately 20 minutes or until golden brown on top.
6. Top with pure maple syrup and berries.

Serves 6

Traditional German Pancake Ingredients
(Inflammatory Foods Highlighted in Bold Italics)
Eggs, *Salt, Sugar, Milk,* Vanilla Extract, *Butter, Unbleached All-Purpose Flour, Vegetable Shortening, Powdered Sugar*

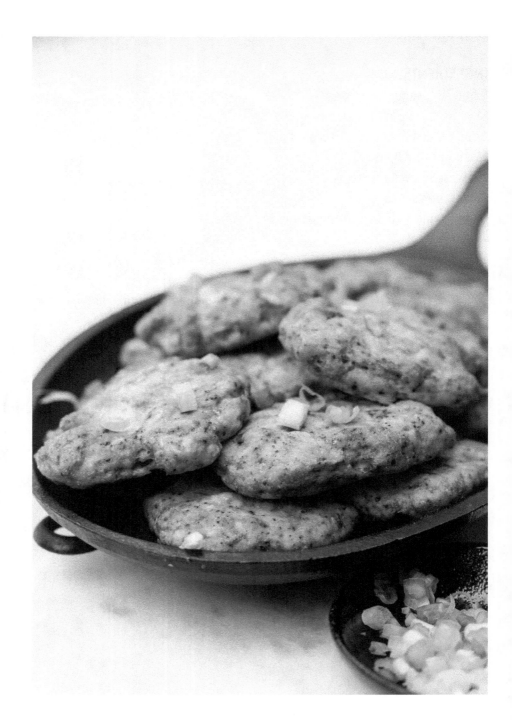

Spicy Turkey Sausage Patties

INGREDIENTS:
2 teaspoons ground ginger
2 pounds raw ground free-range turkey
3 teaspoons black pepper
½ teaspoon cayenne pepper
2 teaspoons dried sage
3/4 teaspoon sea salt
Note: Use less cayenne and or black pepper to reduce the spiciness, as they do have a bit of a kick to them.

INSTRUCTIONS:
1. Preheat oven to 350 degrees.
2. In a large bowl, mix together the ground turkey, ginger, sea salt, sage, cayenne pepper and black pepper until well blended.
3. Grease a cookie sheet with extra virgin olive oil.
4. Grease your hands with extra virgin olive oil (the meat will be very sticky).
5. Form the turkey sausage into 16 patties and lay on a cookie sheet.
6. Bake approximately 11 minutes, turning patties over to brown on both sides, halfway through baking.

Note: You can make this recipe and brown the ground up turkey in a pan, rather than making patties, to use as a topping for the pizza.

Serves approximately 12

Traditional Packaged Breakfast Sausage Ingredients
(Inflammatory Foods Highlighted in Bold Italics)
Corn syrup, potassium lactate, salt, sugar, modified corn starch, monosodium glutamate, sodium diaceate, sodium phosphate, sodium erythorbate, sodium nitrite, and ***natural and artificial flavors,*** collagen casing (potentially inflammatory)

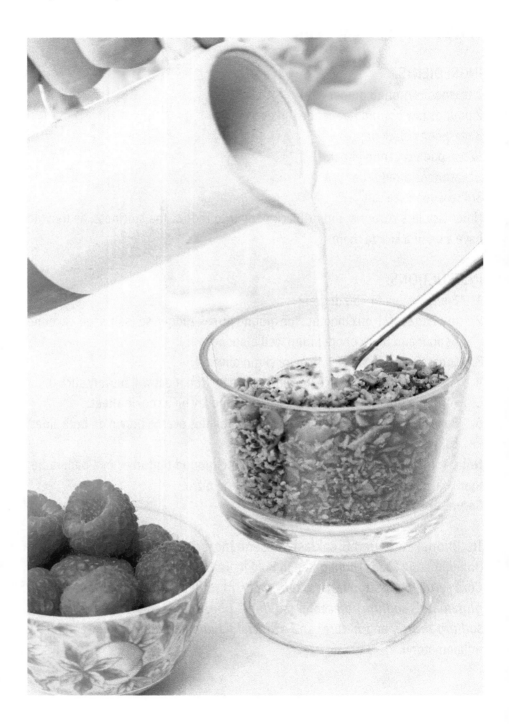

Granola

INGREDIENTS:
1 ½ cups pumpkin seeds
3 cups shredded unsweetened coconut
3/4 cup chia seeds
3/4 cup hemp seeds
3 tablespoons virgin coconut oil
6 tablespoons pure maple syrup
3 teaspoons pumpkin pie spice
½ teaspoon sea salt
1 cup raisins (optional)

INSTRUCTIONS:
1. Preheat oven to 300 degrees.
2. Combine the pumpkin, hemp, and chia seeds in a small food processor, and pulse just enough to break down the seeds into a chunky texture.
3. Transfer seeds to a small bowl and mix in the shredded coconut, coconut oil, maple syrup, pumpkin pie spice, and sea salt.
4. Stir until well coated, then transfer to a baking sheet lined with parchment paper.
5. Spread the mixture out evenly using your hands or a fork.
6. Bake for 20 minutes, stirring half-way through to avoid burning the granola. (You want the mixture nice and golden.)
7. Allow the toasted granola to cool completely, then stir in the raisins and store in an airtight container.
8. Serve with unsweetened almond, hemp, or coconut milk.

Serves 6

Traditional Granola Ingredients
(Inflammatory Foods Highlighted in Bold Italics)
Whole Grain Oats, ***Sugar, Canola Oil,*** Rice Flour, Honey, ***Salt, Brown Sugar Syrup,*** Baking Soda, Soy Lecithin, ***Natural Flavor***

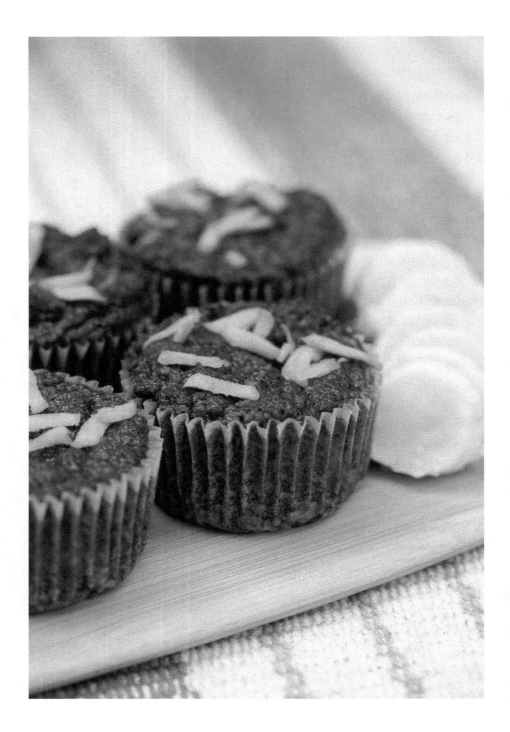

Carrot Banana Bread Muffins

INGREDIENTS:
2 cups almond flour
1 teaspoon apple cider vinegar
¼ teaspoon sea salt
2 teaspoons baking soda
3 fresh medium bananas
1 ½ cups grated carrots
1 tablespoon ground cinnamon
⅛ cup virgin coconut oil
10-12 pitted dates
3 free-range eggs

INSTRUCTIONS:
1. In a small bowl, combine almond flour, baking soda, salt, and cinnamon.
2. In a food processor, combine dates, bananas, eggs, vinegar, and coconut oil. Mix until a smooth, uniform texture appears.
3. Move wet mixture to large bowl and mix in the dry ingredients.
4. Fold in the carrots and walnuts.
5. Spoon mixture into paper-lined muffin tins.
6. Bake at 350 degrees for 25 minutes.

Serves 12 muffins

Traditional Banana Bread Ingredients
(Inflammatory Foods Highlighted in Bold Italics)
Bananas, **Butter,** Baking Soda, **Salt, Granulated Sugar,** Egg, Vanilla Extract, **All Purpose Flour**

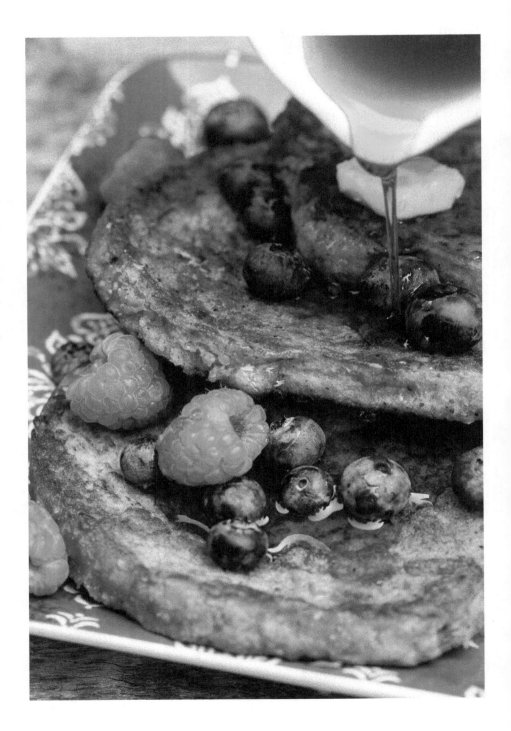

French Toast

INGREDIENTS:
6 eggs
½ cup unsweetened coconut milk
1 tablespoon vanilla extract
½ teaspoon almond extract
Few dashes of nutmeg and cinnamon (I am generous with these to add more flavor)
2 squirts of vanilla crème liquid stevia
6 slices of Ezekiel sprouted bread. Choose gluten-free Ezekiel bread if you want to completely eliminate gluten
Extra virgin coconut oil to grease the pan

INSTRUCTIONS:
1. Warm up your skillet on medium heat and add approximately 1 tablespoon coconut oil.
2. Allow your pan to heat while you make the batter.
3. Mix egg, coconut milk, vanilla, almond extract, nutmeg, cinnamon, and vanilla crème stevia together.
4. Allow bread to soak in mixture for a minute or two on each side.
5. Cook French toast on medium-low heat until it is golden brown on both sides.
6. Top with fresh berries and pure maple syrup or RAW honey.

Serves 6

Traditional French Toast Ingredients
(Inflammatory Foods Highlighted in Bold Italics)
Cinnamon, Nutmeg, *Sugar, Butter,* Eggs, *Milk,* Vanilla Extract, *French Bread*

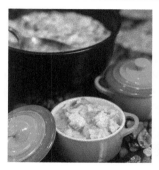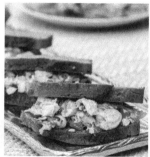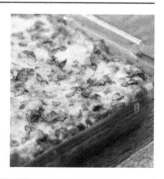

Food Swap Recipes

for Lunch/Dinner

Recipes Free Of: Processed Sugar, Wheat, Cow Dairy, Inflammatory Oils & GMOs

(Be sure to check out the traditional inflammatory foods at the bottom of each recipe, so you can continue to learn what is inflammatory and how to swap those out for non-inflammatory ingredients.)

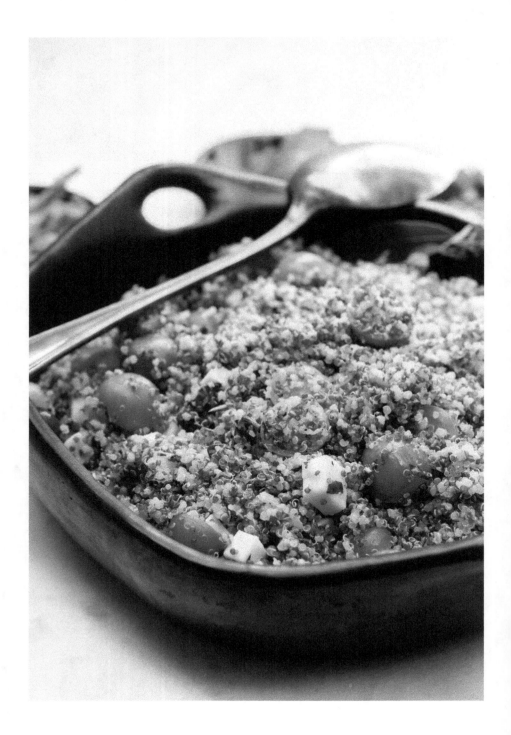

Caprese Quinoa "Pasta" Salad

INGREDIENTS:
2 cups dry quinoa
4 cups water
½ cup fresh lemon juice (about 3 lemons)
¼ cup extra virgin olive oil (the basil-infused extra virgin olive oil from www.genesis-kitchen.com is phenomenal in this recipe)
6 ounces Mt. Sterling Mozzarella Goat Cheese, diced into small cubes
2 packages cherry tomatoes, halved
1 cup fresh basil, chopped into small pieces
2+ teaspoons sea salt, to taste
Black pepper, to taste

INSTRUCTIONS:
1. Combine the 2 cups of dry quinoa with 4 cups of water in a medium saucepan.
2. Over high heat, bring to a boil, then reduce the temperature and cover for 15 minutes, until the quinoa has absorbed all of the water.
3. Fluff with a fork, and allow to cool while you chop the vegetables, cheese, and basil.
4. Mix together lemon juice, olive oil, sea salt, and a dash or two of fresh ground pepper in a large bowl.
5. Add the cooled, cooked quinoa and toss.
6. Combine mozzarella cheese, tomatoes, and fresh basil with the quinoa.
7. Season with additional sea salt and pepper if desired.
8. Serve cold or at room temperature.

Serves 6

Traditional Caprese Pasta Salad Ingredients
(Inflammatory Foods Highlighted in Bold Italics)
Basil, ***Parmesan Cheese,*** Pine Nuts, Garlic, Olive Oil, Cherry Tomatoes, Fresh ***Mozzarella,*** Salt, Pepper, ***Fusilli Pasta***

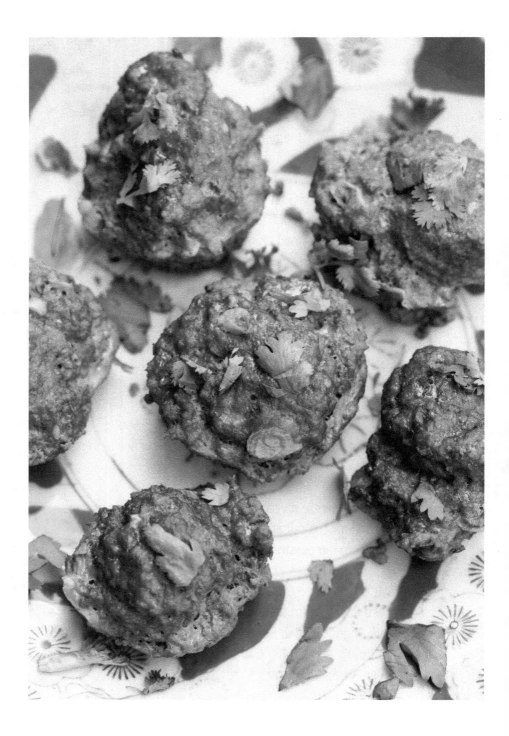

Muffin Tin Meatballs

INGREDIENTS:
4 pounds grass-fed ground beef
3 free-range eggs
1 ½ teaspoons garlic powder
3 teaspoons extra virgin olive oil
3/4 cup green onions
3/4 teaspoon red pepper flakes
3/4 teaspoon sea salt

INSTRUCTIONS:
1. Preheat oven to 375 degrees.
2. Combine ingredients together, thoroughly mixing with your hands.
3. Lightly grease each muffin tin with extra virgin olive oil.
4. Scoop mixture evenly into 24 muffin tins. Place muffin tins on a cookie sheet to catch any juice overflow while cooking.
5. Cook for 30-35 minutes or until golden brown.
6. Allow for meat to cool slightly before serving.

Makes 24 meatballs

NOTE: These meatballs are a great clean protein source. They are easy to pack and delicious to eat alone. Each meatball has approximately 20 grams of protein in it. They are a great protein to help stop cravings in their tracks, as described in Chapter 7.

Traditional Meatball Ingredients
(Inflammatory Foods Highlighted in Bold Italics)
Milk, Breadcrumbs, Egg, *Salt,* Black Pepper, *Parmesan Cheese,* Italian Parsley, *USDA processed meat*

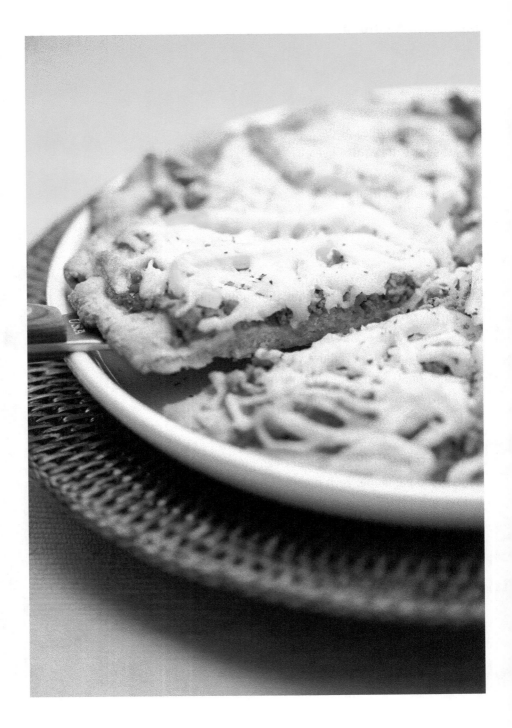

Pizza!

INGREDIENTS:

1 cup water
1 teaspoon granulated garlic
1 ½ cups tapioca flour
½ cup coconut flour

½ cup extra virgin coconut oil
1 ½ teaspoons sea salt
2 free-range eggs

½ jar of Cadia Tomato Basil tomato sauce   (any tomato sauce w/o sugar and citric acid)
2 cups cheese (Manchego sheep cheese, Alta Dena or Goat Mozzarella are great options)
Toppings of choice: Ground "Spicy Turkey Sausage," bell peppers, green onions, mushrooms, red onions, olives, basil, kale, etc.

INSTRUCTIONS:

1. Preheat the oven to 350 degrees. In a medium saucepan, combine coconut oil, water, and sea salt and bring to a boil.
2. Remove from the heat and *immediately* stir in the garlic and tapioca flour.
3. Combine well and let it cool for about 5 minutes. (It should be in a thick ball after adding tapioca.)
4. Next add in the eggs, combining well, and then the coconut flour. Knead the dough until it comes together nicely.
5. Plop the dough onto a parchment-lined cookie sheet and spread it out with your fingers until it is quite thin.
6. Bake for 35 minutes. The bottom should be golden brown when you remove the crust from the oven.
7. Add a thin layer of tomato sauce and toppings. Turn the oven up to broil and bake toppings for 8 minutes or until cheese is thoroughly melted.

NOTE: You can make this and then store in your freezer for frozen pizza. Important note – if freezing, do not melt the cheese or bake for a second time until you are ready to eat it.

Makes approximately 8-10 slices

Traditional Ingredients in Store-Bought Pizza

(Inflammatory Foods Highlighted in Bold Italics)
Mozzarella Cheese, Salt, Modified Food Starch, Cellulose, Milk, Whey Protein, *Natural Flavors, Sodium Propionate,* Tomato Paste, *Sugar,* Spices, *Soybean Oil, Enriched Flour, Maltodextrin, Dextrose, Sodium Stearoyl Lactylate, Calcium Sulfate, Ascorbic Acid,* Yeast

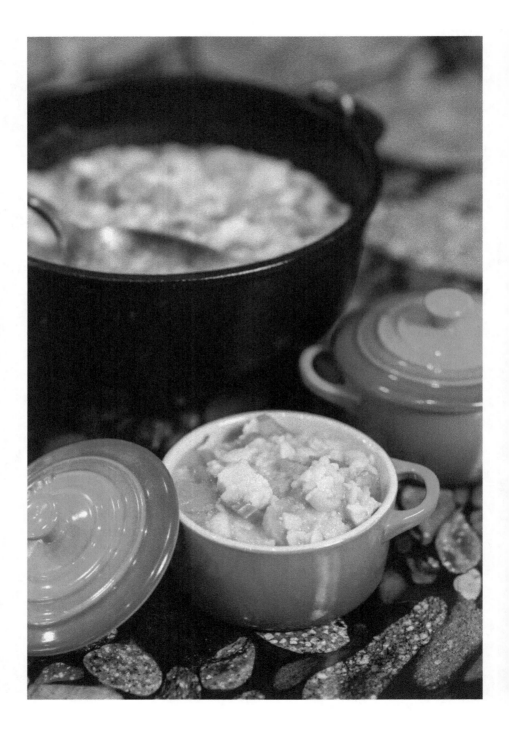

Chicken Noodle Soup

INGREDIENTS:
1 bag of Tinkyada Brown Rice Pasta
1 container of Pacific Organic Bone Broth
5-7 celery stalks
5-7 large organic carrots
Sea salt and pepper to taste
2 pounds organic free-range chicken breast

INSTRUCTIONS:
1. Chop chicken breast into small, bite-size chunks.
2. Combine chicken breast and bone broth into a large pot.
3. Bring chicken and bone broth to a boil, then simmer for approximately 20 minutes or until chicken is cooked through.
4. While chicken is cooking, begin thinly slicing the celery and carrots. Add to the simmering chicken as soon as the vegetables are sliced.
5. Allow the chicken and vegetables to simmer for a good 20 minutes. Add sea salt, pepper, and any additional seasonings you may like.
6. Now, add one bag of Tinkyada pasta to the pot of chicken, bone broth, and vegetables. Allow the pasta to continue simmering (slight boil) for 2 minutes LESS than the directions state on the back of the pasta bag.
7. Remove from heat and add water if you need to adjust the consistency.
8. You can freeze this soup for months at a time. It is great to make an extra-large batch and store in the freezer for those moments you are short on time and need a healthy meal quickly.

Serves 8

Traditional Canned Chicken Noodle Soup Ingredients
(Inflammatory Foods Highlighted in Bold Italics)
Chicken Stock, ***Egg Noodles, USDA Chicken Meat, Salt, Vegetable Oil,*** Potato Starch, ***Monosodium Glutamate, Cane Sugar,*** Water

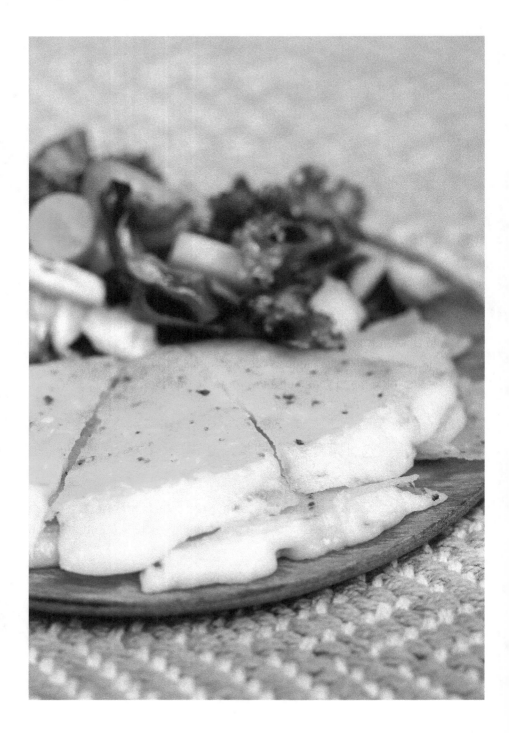

Cheese Quesadilla

INGREDIENTS:

2 Ezekiel tortillas (sprouted wheat or non-GMO sprouted corn are both great options)

2-3 ounces goat cheese (Alta Denta, Mt.Sterling Mozzarella goat cheese, or Manchego sheep cheese are great options)

½ tablespoon coconut oil to grease pan

INSTRUCTIONS:

1. Warm up a pan on medium/medium-high.
2. Grate the cheese of your choice.
3. Place coconut oil in the pan.
4. Sandwich the cheese in-between the two tortillas and then lay in the pan. Add a cover and cook on medium-low until cheese melts and both sides are golden brown.
5. Keep a watchful eye on the quesadillas so as not to burn the tortillas.

Serves 1

Traditional Cheese Quesadilla Ingredients
(Inflammatory Foods Highlighted in Bold Italics)
Flour Tortilla, Butter, Cheese

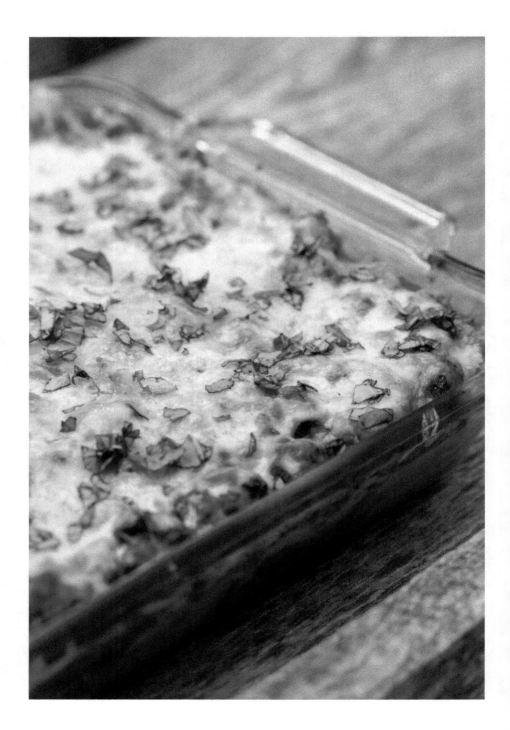

Lasagna

INGREDIENTS:
1 package of Tinkyada Brown Rice lasagna pasta
2-3 packages of Manchego sheep cheese (or sheep/goat cheese of your choice)
1 ½ - 2 lbs. grass fed ground beef
1-2 jars Cadia Basil Tomato sauce (there is no sugar or citric acid in that particular brand AND flavor)
Any additional veggies you may want to add such as bell peppers, onion, spinach, etc.

INSTRUCTIONS:
1. Cook the lasagna noodles for 5 minutes less than stated on the Tinkyada lasagna noodles.
2. Brown the grass-fed ground beef while noodles are cooking.
3. Grate cheese while pasta is cooking.
4. Place noodles (in layers) on parchment paper or tinfoil once they are cooked to eliminate sticking.
5. Alternate meat, cheese, sauce, and pasta to create the lasagna.
6. Cook at 350 degrees for approximately 40 minutes or until cheese bubbles on top.

Serves 12

Traditional Lasagna Ingredients
(Inflammatory Foods Highlighted in Bold Italics)
Olive Oil, ***USDA Ground Beef,*** Onion, Bell Pepper, Garlic, ***Tomato Sauce (typically with sugar),*** tomato paste, crushed tomatoes, oregano, parsley, Italian seasoning, vinegar, ***sugar, salt, lasagna noodles, ricotta cheese, mozzarella cheese, parmesan cheese***

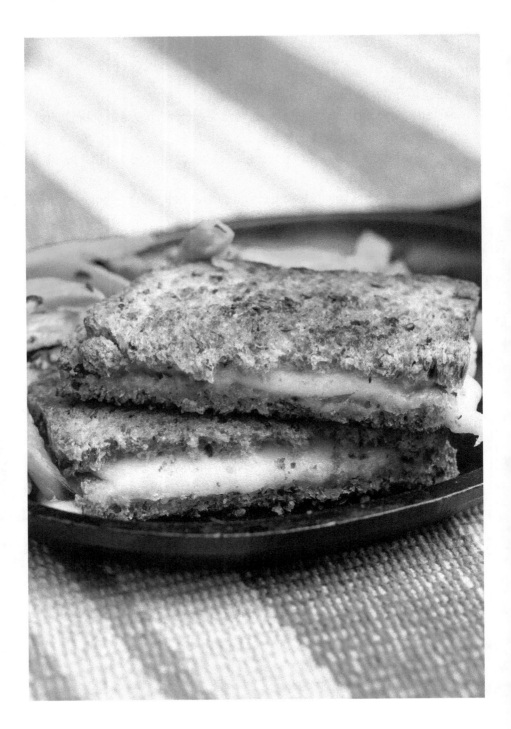

Grilled Cheese Sandwich

INGREDIENTS:
Gluten-Free or Sprouted Wheat Ezekiel Bread
Grate-able and melt-able sheep or goat cheese of your choice (I like Manchego, Alta Dena, or Mt. Sterling cheeses)
Coconut Oil

INSTRUCTIONS:
1. Grate cheese.
2. Add cheese to the bread of your choice.
3. Place coconut oil or grass-fed butter in a pan on medium heat.
4. Place the sandwich in the pan, reduce heat to low, and cover with a lid.
5. Remove from pan once both sides of bread are golden and cheese is melted.

Makes one sandwich

Traditional Grilled Cheese Sandwich Ingredients
(Inflammatory Foods Highlighted in Bold Italics)
Cow Butter, Bread, Cow Cheese

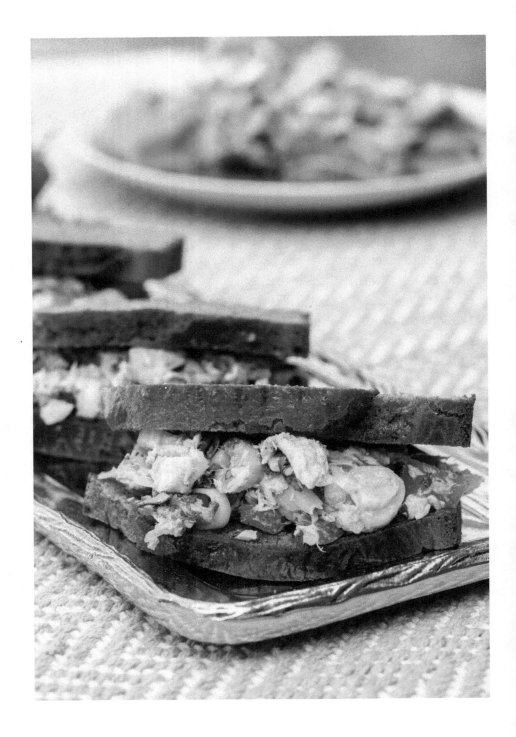

Salmon Avocado Salad Sandwich

INGREDIENTS:

2 pounds wild-caught salmon

2-3 avocados

2-3 tablespoons fresh lemon juice

2 cloves garlic, minced

2 red or yellow bell pepper (be sure to buy organic bell peppers to avoid high pesticide content)

1 small bunch Italian parsley, chopped

1 fennel bulb, sliced thinly

Sea salt and pepper to taste

2 teaspoons ground turmeric

1 teaspoon red pepper flakes

2 cups celery, thinly sliced

1 bunch finely sliced green onion

OPTIONAL: chopped kale and halved cherry tomatoes

To make a sandwich, use the Best Grain-Free Sandwich Bread (at the beginning of these recipes)

INSTRUCTIONS:

1. Bake salmon at 400 degrees for approximately 30 minutes.
2. While salmon is cooking, pit and remove meat of avocados. Place into a medium bowl.
3. Mash avocados with a fork to create a mostly smooth texture.
4. Add lemon juice and garlic. Mix thoroughly.
5. Chop and add all additional vegetables and spices.
6. Once salmon is cooked, allow it to cool slightly.
7. Chop salmon into bite-size pieces and add to avocado mixture.
8. Lay salmon salad over a bed of lettuce, in a cabbage leaf wrap, a sprouted Ezekiel tortilla, or – my favorite – on top of a slice of the Best Grain-Free Sandwich Bread.

Serves 8

Traditional Tuna Salad Sandwich Ingredients

(Inflammatory Foods Highlighted in Bold Italics)

Tuna (fish) Meat, Celery, Red Onion, Parsley, ***Mayonnaise,*** Mustard, Black Pepper, Lemon Juice, ***Salt***

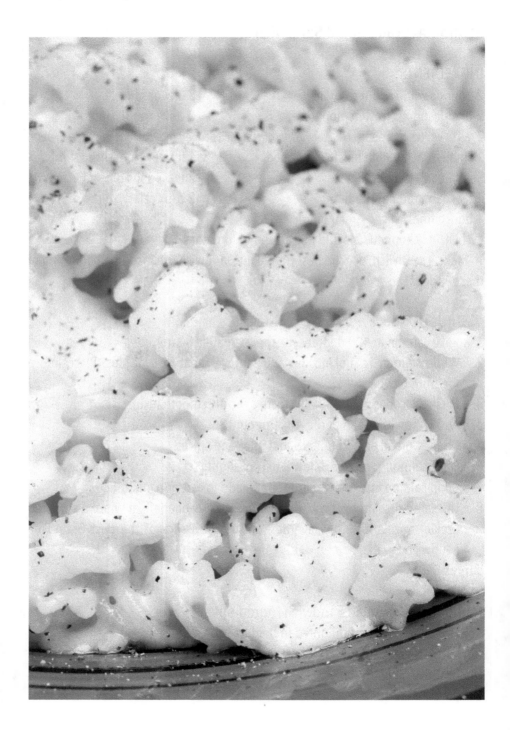

Mac 'N' Cheese

INGREDIENTS:

1 bag Tinkyada brown rice pasta (you can play with shells or spirals)
6 ounces of a shreddable and meltable goat cheese: Alta Dena Goat, Mt. Sterling Goat, or Manchego Sheep Cheese are great options
Sea salt and pepper to taste

INSTRUCTIONS:

1. Follow cooking directions on the bag of Tinkyada pasta (takes approximately 14 minutes).
2. While pasta is cooking, grate cheese.
3. Strain pasta and put back in pot. Immediately add grated cheese.
4. Gently mix cheese and pasta together so the cheese melts.
5. Add sea salt and pepper to taste.

Serves 4

Note: No need to add milk or butter, as this cheese is quite rich and delicious on its own.

Traditional Mac 'N' Cheese Ingredients

(Inflammatory Foods Highlighted in Bold Italics)

Macaroni Pasta, Cheese Sauce, Salt, Sodium Tripolyphosphate, Citric Acid, Lactic Acid, Sodium Phosphate, Calcium Phosphate

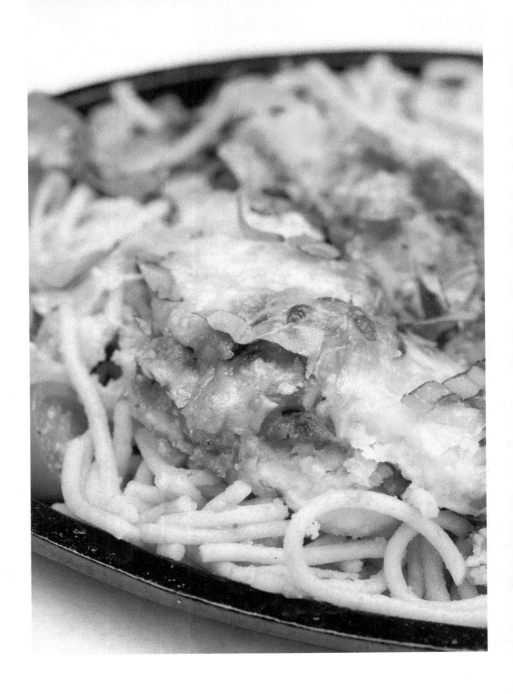

Chicken Parmesan

INGREDIENTS:

1 ½ pounds of free-range boneless, skinless, chicken breasts (or strips for the Chicken Fingers variation)

½ cup coconut flour (or almond flour)   ½ tablespoon garlic powder

3 free-range eggs

1 jar Cadia Tomato Basil sauce (or any tomato sauce without sugar)

2 cups grated Manchego sheep cheese (optional)

Coconut Oil for frying

1 package of Tinkyada brown rice spaghetti pasta

1 teaspoon dried basil   1 teaspoon sea salt

½ teaspoon garlic powder   ½ teaspoon oregano

INSTRUCTIONS:

1. Put 2-3 tablespoons of coconut oil in a large skillet and turn on medium heat.
2. Slice each chicken breast length-wise, making each strip approximately ½ inch thick.
3. Beat eggs in a medium-sized bowl.
4. On a large plate or dish, combine coconut flour and spices.
5. Dip the chicken into the egg mixture and then into the flour mixture until well coated.
6. Place chicken directly into hot oil and cook, flipping once, until both sides have browned and chicken is cooked (about 2-4 minutes per side).
7. While chicken is cooking, heat sauce over medium heat until warmed, and cook Tinkyada brown rice pasta on the stove (app. 14 minutes).
8. Layer pasta then chicken and tomato sauce.
9. Add cheese and broil for a few minutes or until cheese is melted.

Serves 8

Traditional Chicken Parmesan Ingredients

(Inflammatory Foods Highlighted in Bold Italics)

USDA Chicken, Salt, Eggs, ***Breadcrumbs, Parmesan Cheese,*** Olive Oil, Basil, ***Mozzarella Cheese***

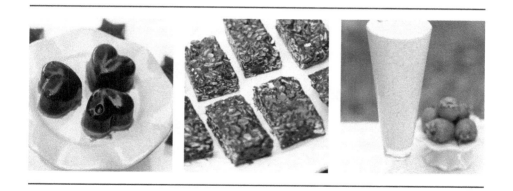

Food Swap Recipes

for Snacks

Recipes Free Of: Processed Sugar, Wheat, Cow Dairy, Inflammatory Oils & GMOs

(Be sure to check out the traditional inflammatory foods at the bottom of each recipe, so you can continue to learn what is inflammatory and how to swap those out for non-inflammatory ingredients.)

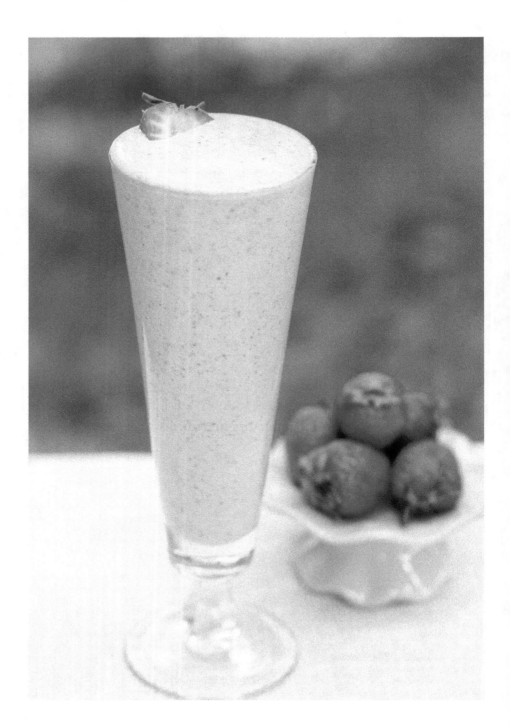

Strawberry Protein Milkshake

INGREDIENTS:
6 ounces frozen strawberries
1-2 scoops vanilla protein powder without processed sugar (Sun Warrior Classic version is a good brand)
½ cup of unsweetened vanilla coconut, almond, or hemp milk
2 tablespoons unsweetened almond butter

INSTRUCTIONS:
1. Combine all ingredients into blender.
2. Add more or less milk depending on desired thickness.
3. Blend until smooth.
Serves 1 large smoothie

Traditional Strawberry Milkshake Ingredients
(Inflammatory Foods Highlighted in Bold Italics)
Whole Milk, Vanilla Extract, Strawberries, ***Vanilla Ice Cream***

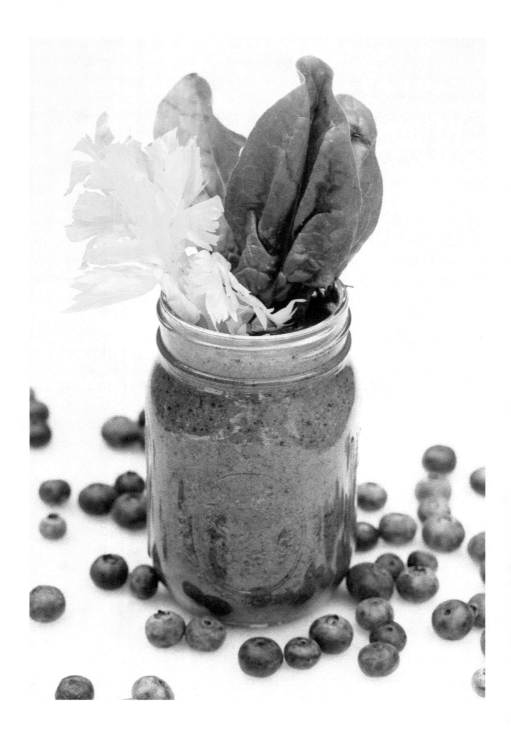

Green Detox Smoothie

INGREDIENTS:
1 organic cucumber
2-3 cups chopped kale or dark leafy greens
Juice from 1 lemon
½ to 1 whole avocado
2 scoops protein powder (I typically use vanilla)
⅓ cup hemp seeds
½ cup frozen organic berries

INSTRUCTIONS:
1.   Blend all ingredients together, adding the protein powder last.
Serves 1 large smoothie

Traditional Green Detox Smoothie Ingredients
(Inflammatory Foods Highlighted in Bold Italics)
Typically green detox smoothies are free of inflammation. Be sure to make sure any supplement or protein powder used is free of the top inflammatory foods, especially processed sugar.

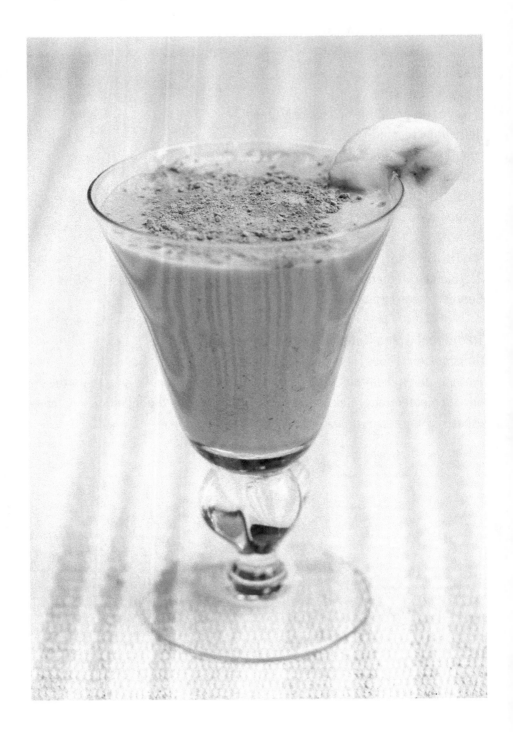

Chocolate Banana Split Protein Milkshake

INGREDIENTS:
1 ½ medium to large bananas
1-2 scoops chocolate protein powder without processed sugar (such as Sun Warrior Classic version)
½ cup of unsweetened coconut, almond, or hemp milk
1 dropper of vanilla crème liquid stevia
Handful of ice cubes

INSTRUCTIONS:
1. Combine all ingredients into a blender.
2. Add more or less milk to desired thickness.
Serves 1 large smoothie

Traditional Chocolate Milkshake Ingredients
(Inflammatory Foods Highlighted in Bold Italics)
Ice cream, Chocolate Syrup, Milk

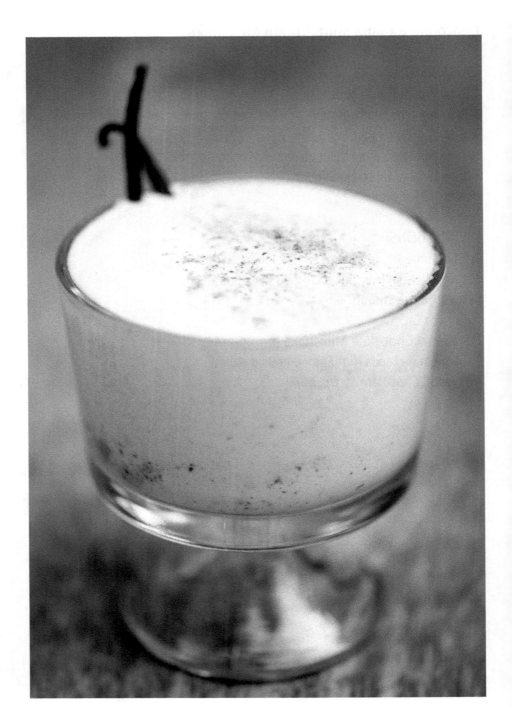

Blended Chai Protein Smoothie

INGREDIENTS:
1 cup light or regular unsweetened canned coconut milk
1-2 scoops vanilla protein powder (I like Vanilla Sun Warrior CLASSIC protein powder)
1 teaspoon vanilla extract
½ rounded teaspoon pumpkin pie spice
15 drops vanilla crème liquid stevia
½ avocado
1 handful of ice

INSTRUCTIONS:
1. Combine all ingredients into a blender.
2. Blend on high until smoothie is smooth and fluffy.
3. Enjoy – this is one of my favorite smoothies!
Makes 1 large smoothie

Traditional Blended Chai Ingredients
(Inflammatory Foods Highlighted in Bold Italics)
Milk, Crème Frappuccino Syrup, Sugar, Natural and Artificial Flavor, Xanthan Gum, Citric Acid, Chai Tea Concentrate

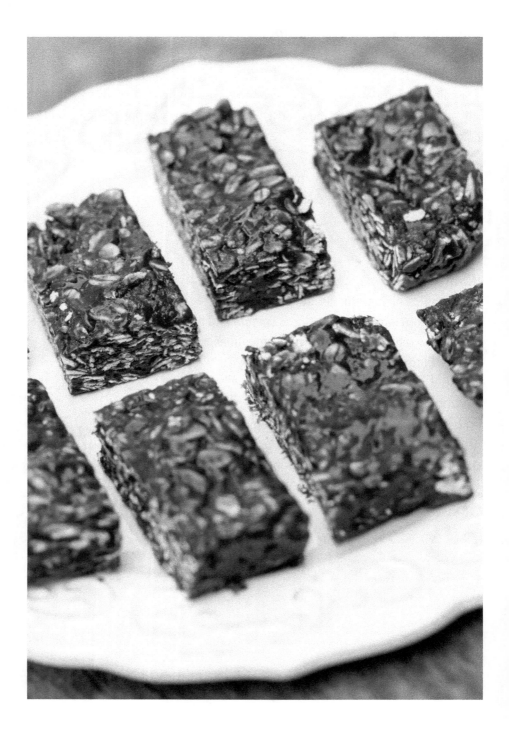

Classic Granola Bars

INGREDIENTS:
2 cups gluten-free rolled oats
½ cup creamy unsweetened almond or sun butter
⅓ cup honey
½ teaspoon sea salt
1 teaspoon cinnamon
4 tablespoons raw cacao powder (optional for a more chocolatey flavor)

INSTRUCTIONS:
1. Line a standard loaf pan with parchment paper and set aside.
2. In a small saucepan over medium-high heat, bring honey to a boil. Set a timer, and allow the honey to continue boiling for one minute.
3. In the meantime, place the oats in a large bowl and set aside.
4. Remove the pan of honey from the heat and stir in the nut/seed butter, cinnamon, cacao powder, and sea salt.
5. Immediately pour the warm honey mixture over the oats, and use a spatula to stir well, coating the oats evenly. As the mixture cools, it will become sticky and difficult to mix, so be sure to move quickly!
6. Transfer the mixture to the lined bread loaf pan and press HARD to pack it into the pan. Pressing firmly will ensure the bars stick together well later.
7. Place the pan in the fridge or freezer to cool, then use a large knife to cut the bars.

Makes 12 bars

Traditional Granola Bar Ingredients
(Inflammatory Foods Highlighted in Bold Italics)
Whole Rolled Oats, ***Brown Sugar, Crisp Rice, Soybean Oil, Whole Wheat Flour, Sodium Bicarbonate, Soy*** Lecithin, ***Caramel Color, Nonfat Dry Milk, Corn Syrup***

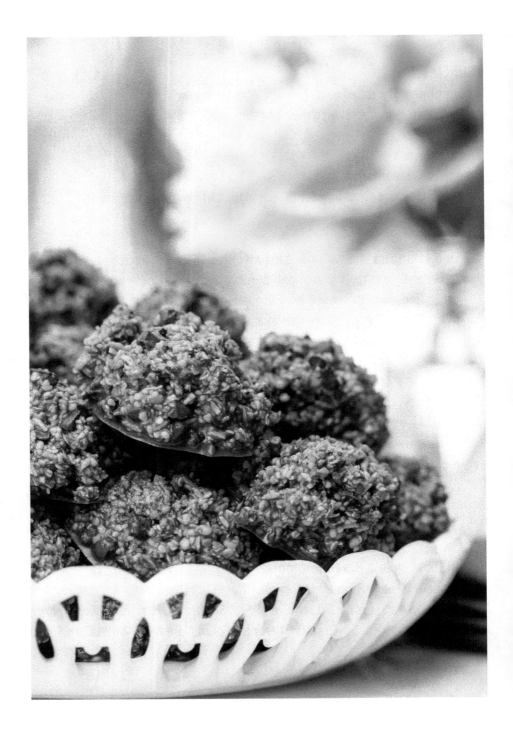

Hemp Chocolate Joy Balls

INGREDIENTS:
3/4 cup cacao nibs
1 3/4 cups unsweetened shredded coconut meat
1 ½ cups softened coconut oil
2 cups shelled organic hemp seeds
4 tablespoons raw honey
7 scoops chocolate protein powder (Find a clean protein powder like the Sun Warrior Classic brand, without any processed sugar.)

INSTRUCTIONS:
1. Soften the coconut oil and mix everything together – it will be slightly crumbly (depending on how soft the coconut oil is).
2. *Tightly* squish the mixture together into balls and place in a storage container.
3. Store and freezer and remove when ready to eat. Great snack for traveling!

Makes 44 chocolate balls

Traditional Hemp Chocolate Joy Ball Ingredients
(Inflammatory Foods Highlighted in Bold Italics)
There are no inflammatory ingredients here … a unique recipe full of omega-3 fats and rich in antioxidants.

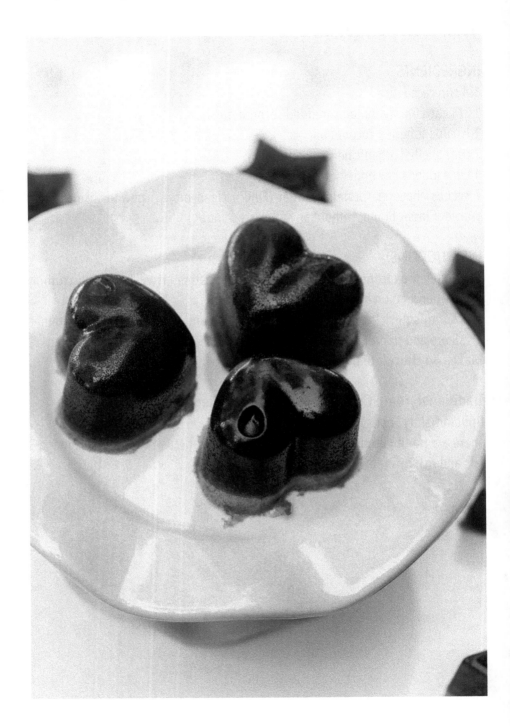

Protein Fruit Gummies

INGREDIENTS:
1 3/4 cups raw coconut water
2 cups unsweetened organic frozen cherries (pitted)
6 full squirts of vanilla crème liquid stevia
½ cup grass-fed gelatin (I like Great Lakes Collagen Gelatin)
½ teaspoon almond extract

INSTRUCTIONS:
1. Place the coconut water, almond extract, and frozen cherries in a blender on high until completely mixed.
2. Pour mixture into a saucepan.
3. Add stevia and gelatin. Whisk together. The gelatin will be clumpy at first.
4. Turn the heat on low and continue to whisk for 5-10 minutes, until it becomes thin and everything is incorporated.
5. Remove from heat.
6. Pour into silicone molds or a small baking dish. Set in the refrigerator for at least one hour to firm up.
7. If you used a small baking dish, cut into bite-size squares or cut out shapes using a cookie cutter.

Makes 24 bite-sized gummies

Traditional Fruit Gummies Ingredients
(Inflammatory Foods Highlighted in Bold Italics)
Fruit Puree, *Corn Syrup, Sugar, Modified Corn Starch,* Gelatin, *Citric Acid, Lactic Acid, Natural and Artificial Flavors,* Ascorbic Acid, Alpha Tocopherol Acetate, *Sodium Citrate,* Coconut Oil, *Caranuba Wax, Annatto Color, Red 40, Blue 1*

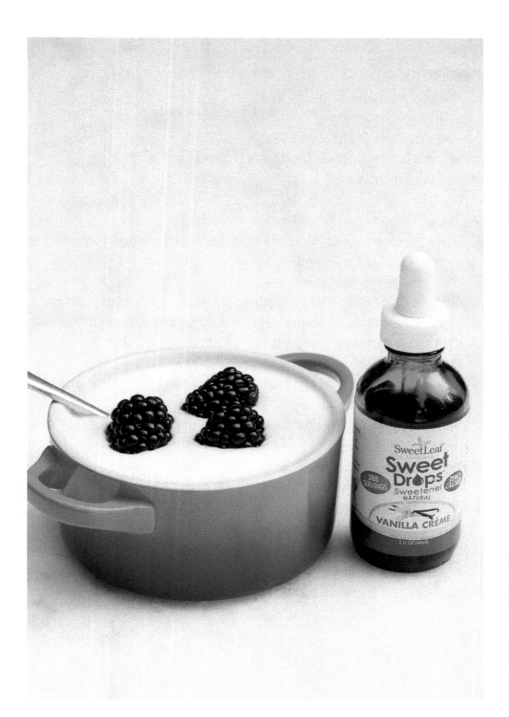

Flavored Yogurt (Vanilla Crème or Berry)

INGREDIENTS:
6 oz. Bellewether PLAIN sheep yogurt OR any plain goat yogurt
1-2 squirts liquid stevia (vanilla crème or berry)
Fresh berries to top

INSTRUCTIONS:
1.   Mix yogurt with liquid stevia.
2.   Top with fresh berries.
Serves 1

Traditional Vanilla Yogurt Ingredients
(Inflammatory Foods Highlighted in Bold Italics)
Reduced Fat Milk, Sugar, Modified Corn Starch, Kosher Gelatin, ***Natural Flavor,***
Yogurt Cultures, Vitamin D

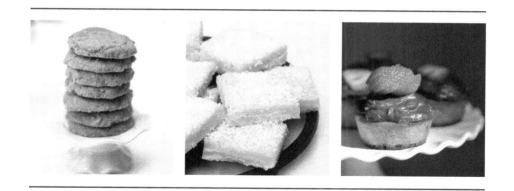

Food Swap Recipes

for Dessert

Recipes Free Of: Processed Sugar, Wheat, Cow Dairy, Inflammatory Oils & GMOs

(Be sure to check out the traditional inflammatory foods at the bottom of each recipe, so you can continue to learn what is inflammatory and how to swap those out for non-inflammatory ingredients.)

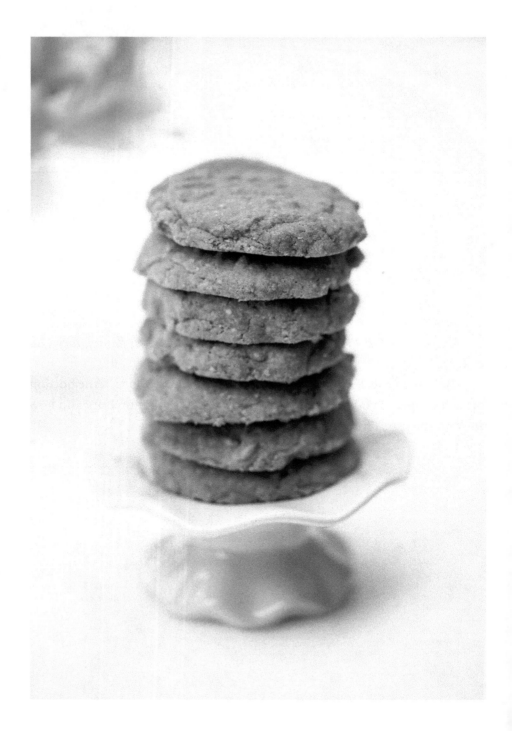

Ginger Molasses Cookies

INGREDIENTS:
1 ½ cups almond flour
2 tablespoons coconut oil, softened
¼ cup pure maple syrup
1 tablespoon blackstrap molasses
2 teaspoons ground ginger
⅛ teaspoon fine sea salt
¼ teaspoon baking soda

INSTRUCTIONS:
1. Preheat the oven to 350 degrees.
2. Combine all of the ingredients in a medium bowl and mix until a thick batter is formed.
3. Drop the batter by rounded tablespoons onto a baking sheet lined with wax paper or parchment paper. Use a wet fork to flatten each dough mound, to your desired cookie thickness.
4. Bake for 8-10 minutes, until firm around the edges but still soft in the center.
5. Allow to cool on the pan for 10 minutes before transferring to rack to cool completely.

Serves 12

Traditional Ginger Molasses Cookie Ingredients
(Inflammatory Foods Highlighted in Bold Italics)
All Purpose Flour, Ginger, Baking Soda, Cinnamon, Cloves, ***Salt, Margarine, Sugar,*** Egg, Water, ***Molasses***

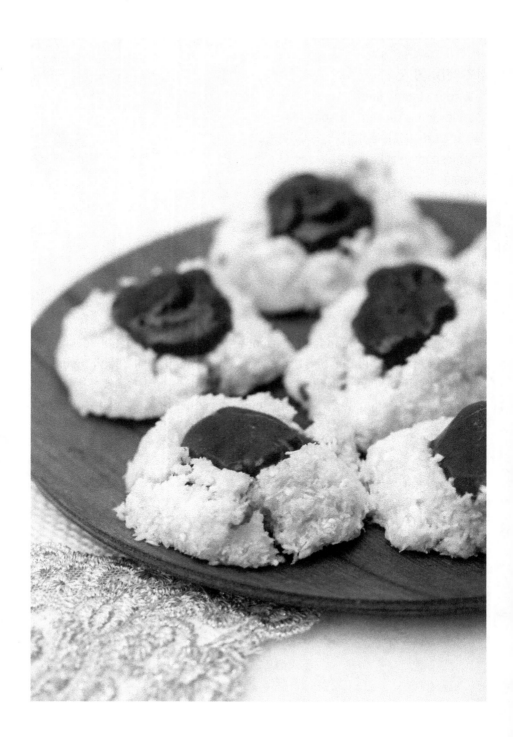

Vanilla Chocolate Kisses

INGREDIENTS:

For the Vanilla Cookies

2 cups shredded unsweetened coconut

6 tablespoons maple syrup

2 teaspoons vanilla extract

4 tablespoons softened coconut oil

a pinch of salt

For the Chocolate Kisses

4 tablespoons coconut oil, softened

2 tablespoons raw cacao powder

A few grains of salt

2 tablespoons pure maple syrup

INSTRUCTIONS:

1. Line cookie tray with parchment paper.
2. Mix all vanilla cookie ingredients together by hand.
3. Scoop dough into tablespoon-sized balls and place on parchment paper.
4. Place in the fridge for 5 minutes while you prepare the chocolate filling.
5. Combine everything for chocolate kisses in a food processor.
6. Set aside in the refrigerator to cool for 5-10 minutes.
7. Remove the coconut balls from the fridge and gently press down in the middle of each cookie to create an indentation.
8. Remove chocolate from refrigerator.
9. Carefully spoon the chocolate into each indentation.
10. Return to the fridge for 5 minutes or until the chocolate sets.

Serves 15

Note: Cookies are best stored in the refrigerator or freezer.

Traditional "Almond Joy" Ingredients

(Inflammatory Foods Highlighted in Bold Italics)

Sweetened Condensed Milk, Vanilla Extract, S***alt, Confectioners Sugar, Sweetened Flaked Coconut,*** Almonds, ***Milk Chocolate***

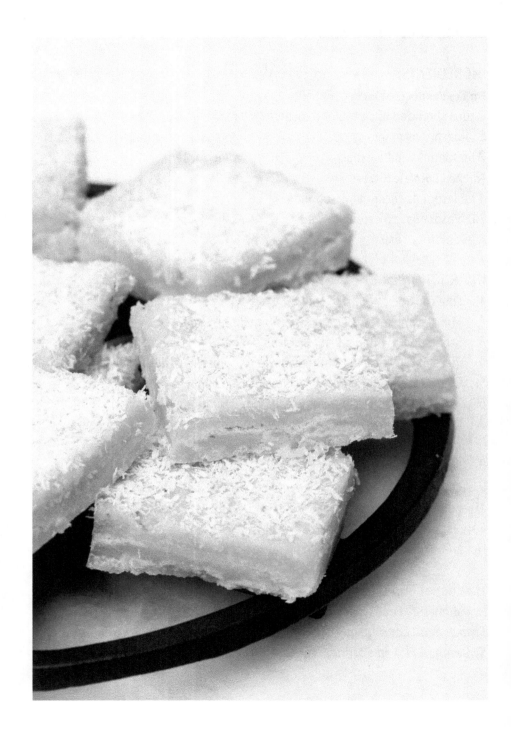

Zesty Lemon Bar

INGREDIENTS:

For Filling:

4 tablespoons lemon-infused extra virgin olive oil (from www.genesis-kitchen.com) or coconut oil

4 tablespoons of raw honey   1 ½ cups almond flour

½ cup fresh lemon juice   ½ cup unsweetened finely shredded coconut flakes

3 eggs   (to spread on top of the filling once cooked)

For Crust:

2 tablespoons lemon infused extra virgin olive oil or coconut oil

1 tablespoon raw honey   1 teaspoon pure vanilla extract

INSTRUCTIONS:

1. Preheat the oven to 350 degrees.
2. Grease 8" square baking dish and dust with almond flour.
3. In bowl, whisk together 2 tablespoons oil, 1 tablespoon raw honey, and vanilla.
4. Stir the wet ingredients into the almond flour until thoroughly combined and press the dough into the prepared dish.
5. Bake for 15-17 minutes until lightly golden.
6. While baking crust, prepare the topping.
7. In a blender combine the other 4 tablespoons of oil, 4 tablespoons of honey, eggs, and lemon juice. Process on high until smooth.
8. Remove crust from oven and pour the topping evenly over the *hot* crust.
9. Bake for 15-20 minutes until the topping is golden.
10. Sprinkle with unsweetened, finely shredded coconut flakes.
11. Let cool in the dish for 30 minutes then refrigerate for 2 hours to set.
12. Cut into bars and serve.

Serves 12

Traditional Lemon Bar Ingredients

(Inflammatory Foods Highlighted in Bold Italics)

Flour, Butter, Powdered Sugar, Granulated Sugar, Lemon Peel, Lemon Juice, Baking Powder, ***Salt,*** Egg

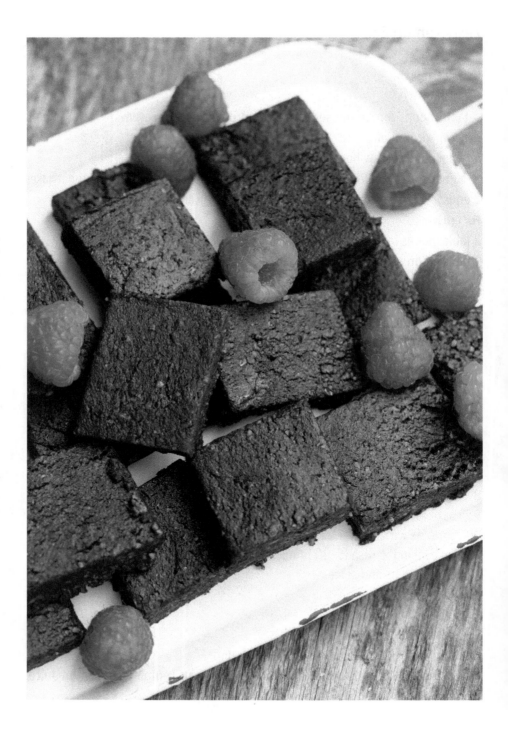

Carr Family Brownie

INGREDIENTS:
1 cup cacao powder
16 pitted Medjool dates
1 teaspoon vanilla extract
½ teaspoon sea salt
3 cups raw walnuts
Filtered water

INSTRUCTIONS:
1. Place the walnuts and salt in a food processor.
2. Add the dates, cacao powder, and vanilla.
3. Process until the mixture begins to stick together.
4. Add one teaspoon of water at a time to give the brownies just enough moisture to make the dough stick together.
5. Press dough into a baking dish and chill for 2 hours.
Serves 16

Traditional Brownie Ingredients
(Inflammatory Foods Highlighted in Bold Italics)
Dark Chocolate, Butter, Sugar, Egg, Vanilla Extract, ***Flour,*** Cocoa Powder, ***Salt***

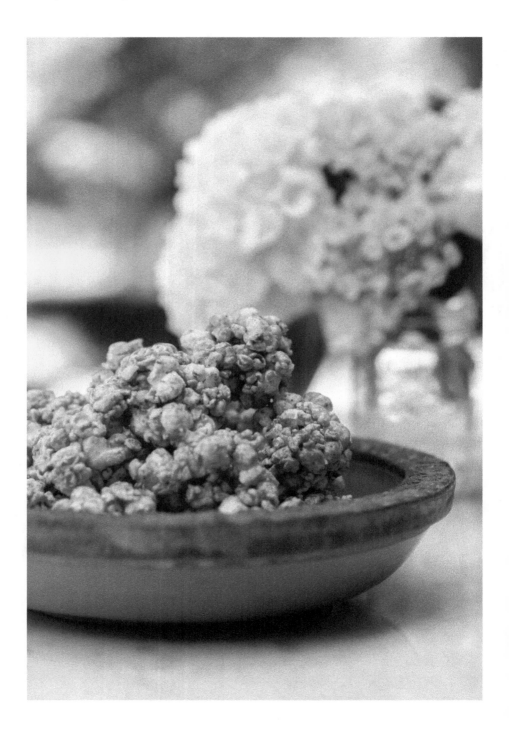

Popcorn Balls

INGREDIENTS:

½ cup almond butter or sun butter (unsweetened)
½ cup raw honey
5 tablespoons coconut oil
1 teaspoon sea salt

2 tablespoons vanilla extract
½ cup non-GMO popcorn kernels

INSTRUCTIONS:

1. Pop popcorn by adding 2 tablespoons coconut oil to ½ cup non-GMO popcorn kernels in a large pot. Cover and cook on high. As popping begins to slow down, remove from heat so as not to burn the bottom of the popcorn.
2. Add almond or sun butter, raw honey, sea salt, and vanilla extract to a large pot over medium heat. Stir the mixture to combine.
3. Allow the mixture to heat until it just begins to bubble then turn the heat down. Simmer on low heat for another 2-3 minutes.
4. Line a cookie sheet with parchment paper.
5. Remove mixture from heat and add all the popcorn.
6. Using a long handled wooden spoon, stir the popcorn and almond butter mixture until all the popcorn is coated.
7. Allow popcorn to cool so you can touch it without burning your hands.
8. Oil your hands with coconut oil so mixture will not stick to them.
9. Pick up a palm full of popcorn and form it into a tight ball.
10. Place the ball on the parchment paper and allow to cool. As it cools, it will continue to harden.
11. Repeat for all popcorn balls.

Makes 12 balls

Traditional Popcorn Ball Ingredients

(Inflammatory Foods Highlighted in Bold Italics)

Light Corn Syrup, Margarine, Water, ***Confectioners Sugar, Marshmallows, Plain Popcorn***

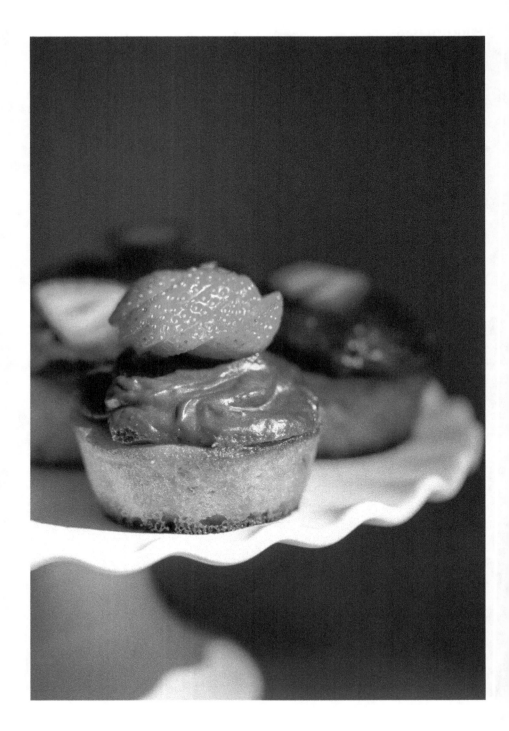

Vanilla Cupcakes with Chocolate Avocado Frosting

INGREDIENTS:

For Cake:
½ cup coconut flour
¼ teaspoon sea salt
¼ teaspoon baking soda
6 large eggs
½ cup virgin coconut oil
4 tablespoons pure maple syrup
2 tablespoons vanilla extract

For Chocolate Avocado Frosting:
3 tablespoons extra virgin coconut oil
1 extra large avocado
4 ½ tablespoons cacao powder
⅓ cup raw honey

INSTRUCTIONS:

For Cake:
1. In a food processor, combine coconut flour, salt, and baking soda.
2. Add eggs, coconut oil, maple syrup, and vanilla.
3. Line a cupcake pan with 12 paper liners and scoop ¼ cup into each.
4. Bake at 350 degrees for 20-24 minutes.
5. Cool for 1 hour.

For Frosting:
1. Process all ingredients in a food processor (or high-quality blender) until smooth.
2. Let the frosting cool for a few minutes before icing the cake.

Makes 12 cupcakes

Traditional Vanilla Cupcake Ingredients
(Inflammatory Foods Highlighted in Bold Italics)
All Purpose Flour, Baking Powder, ***Salt, Sugar, Butter,*** Egg, Vanilla Extract, ***Milk***

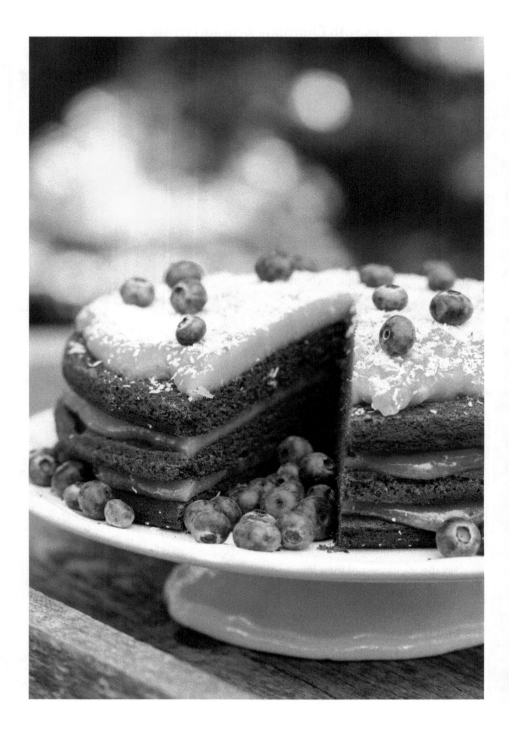

Chocolate Cake with Vanilla Frosting

INGREDIENTS:

For Cake:

½ teaspoon baking soda
12 free-range eggs
1 cup virgin coconut oil
½ cup raw cacao powder

1 cup coconut flour
1 cup pure maple syrup
4 tablespoons vanilla extract
1 teaspoon salt

For Vanilla Icing:

2 cans of full-fat coconut cream (liquid drained from can)
4 tablespoons pure maple syrup   4 teaspoons vanilla extract
½ teaspoon almond extract

INSTRUCTIONS:

For Cake:

1. Add all of the ingredients to a blender and blend on high for 30-45 seconds, allowing the eggs to froth.
2. Pour batter evenly into two 6 inch cake pans.
3. Bake at 350 degrees for 30 minutes or until cake passes the toothpick test.
4. Cool before frosting.

For Vanilla Icing:

1. Chill coconut milk in the fridge for at least 6 hours, preferably overnight. (Recipe will not work without it being chilled.)
2. Without shaking the cans, remove them from the refrigerator.
3. Carefully open the cans of coconut milk and scoop the thickened cream into a bowl.
4. Add the pure maple syrup, vanilla extract, and almond extract to the heavy coconut cream.
5. Mix thoroughly with a hand mixer... will take 3-5 minutes.
6. Place in refrigerator and allow icing to cool to thicken until it meets the texture you most prefer. Frost the cake.

Makes two-layer 6" cake

Traditional Chocolate Cake Ingredients

(Inflammatory Foods Highlighted in Bold Italics)

Butter, Egg, ***Sugar, Flour,*** Cocoa Powder, Baking Soda, Baking Powder, Vanilla, ***Milk***

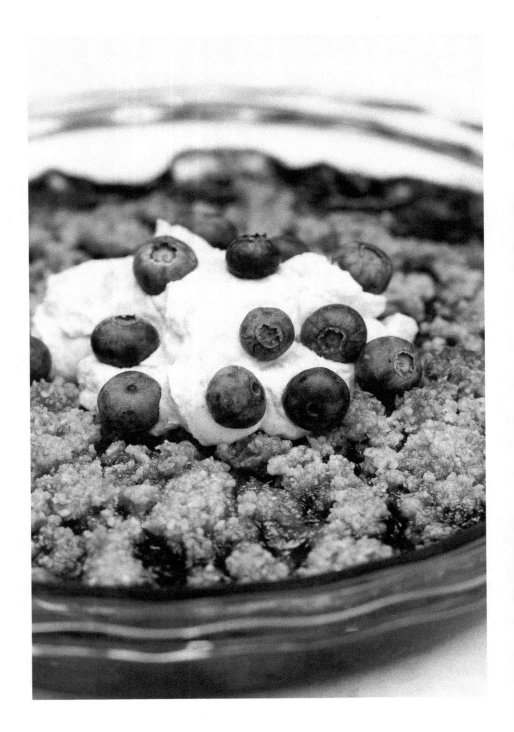

Blueberry Peach Cobbler

INGREDIENTS:
Filling:
2 pounds organic or freshly thawed from frozen peaches, roughly chopped
2 cups organic fresh or frozen blueberries
¼ cup pure maple syrup   1 teaspoon vanilla extract
½ teaspoon ground cinnamon
Crumb Topping:
1 ½ cups walnut halves   ½ cup shredded unsweetened coconut
2 tablespoons pure maple syrup   1 tablespoon melted coconut oil
¼ teaspoon sea salt

INSTRUCTIONS:
1. Preheat oven to 350 degrees.
2. In a large saucepan, over medium heat, combine the peaches, blueberries, maple syrup, vanilla, and ground cinnamon. Stir until the syrup comes to a boil, then allow mixture to simmer until the syrup has thickened a bit and the peaches are fork tender. Turn off the heat and allow the pot to sit while you make the crumble.
3. To make the crumble, place the walnuts and shredded coconut in the bowl of a large food processor. Process until a crumbly texture is formed, then add the maple syrup, coconut oil, sea salt, and almond extract. Process again, until a sticky and crumbly mixture is formed.
4. Pour the peach filling into a 9-inch square or round baking dish, then sprinkle the crumble over the top evenly.
5. Bake at 350 degrees for 15 minutes, or until the top is lightly golden. Serve warm.

Serves 8

Traditional Peach Cobbler Ingredients
(Inflammatory Foods Highlighted in Bold Italics)
Peaches, ***Sugar, Brown Sugar,*** Cinnamon, Nutmeg, Lemon Juice, ***Cornstarch, All Purpose Flour,*** Baking Soda, ***Salt, Butter***

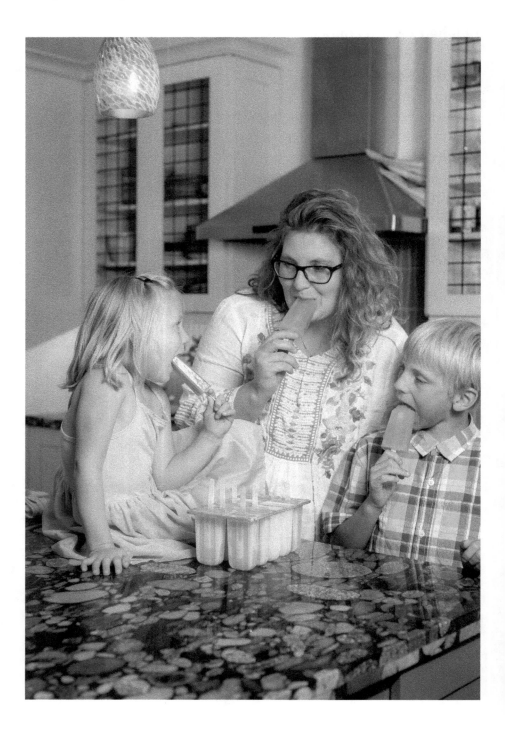

Watermelon Popsicles

INGREDIENTS:
1 ½ cups sliced watermelon
4 reusable Popsicle containers

INSTRUCTIONS:
1. Blend the slices of watermelon in a blender (you may need to add a tiny amount of water to get the watermelon blended).
2. Pour watermelon juice into reusable Popsicle containers.
3. Freeze overnight.

Makes 4

Traditional Fruit Popsicle Ingredients
(Inflammatory Foods Highlighted in Bold Italics)
Fruit Puree, Water, *__Cane Sugar, Juice For Color, Malic Acid, Natural Flavor,__* Guar Gum, *__Ascorbic Acid__*

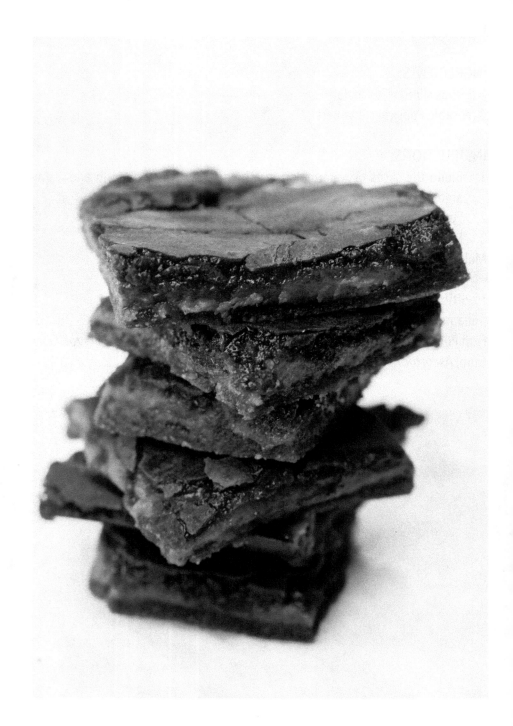

Reese's Almond Butter Chocolate Bars

INGREDIENTS:

For Chocolate Crust:

3/4 cup ground almond meal
2 tablespoons pure maple syrup
Pinch of sea salt

2 tablespoons cocoa powder
1 tablespoon melted coconut oil

For Almond Butter Filling:

½ cup creamy unsweetened almond butter
3 tablespoons pure maple syrup
Generous pinch of sea salt

1 tablespoon melted coconut oil

For Chocolate Topping:

¼ cup cocoa powder
3 tablespoons pure maple syrup

¼ cup melted coconut oil

INSTRUCTIONS:

1. Line a standard 9x12 inch cake pan with parchment paper and set it aside.
2. In a medium bowl, stir together all of the chocolate crust ingredients until a moist dough is formed.
3. Press the dough evenly into the bottom of the lined loaf pan, and place it in the freezer to set.
4. In a medium bowl, stir together the almond butter, maple syrup, coconut oil, and salt.
5. Remove the crust from the freezer and pour the almond butter filling over the top, using a spatula to spread it out evenly.
6. Return the pan to the freezer to set.
7. For the final layer, combine the cocoa powder, melted coconut oil, and maple syrup in a bowl, whisking it well to break up any clumps.
8. Once the mixture has become a smooth chocolate sauce, pour it over the almond butter layer, and return pan to the freezer to set until firm, about an hour or two.
9. Once the bars are firm, grab the edges of parchment paper to easily lift the solid almond butter chocolate bars from the pan. Use a sharp knife to slice the bars into your desired size.
10. Store them in an air-tight container in the fridge for up to two weeks, or in the freezer for up to a month.

Makes 25 bites

Traditional Reese's Peanut Butter Cup Ingredients

(Inflammatory Foods Highlighted in Bold Italics)

Milk Chocolate, Peanuts, Dextrose, Cocoa Butter, ***Partially Hydrogenated Vegetable Oil,*** Salt, ***Emulsifier, Preservative***

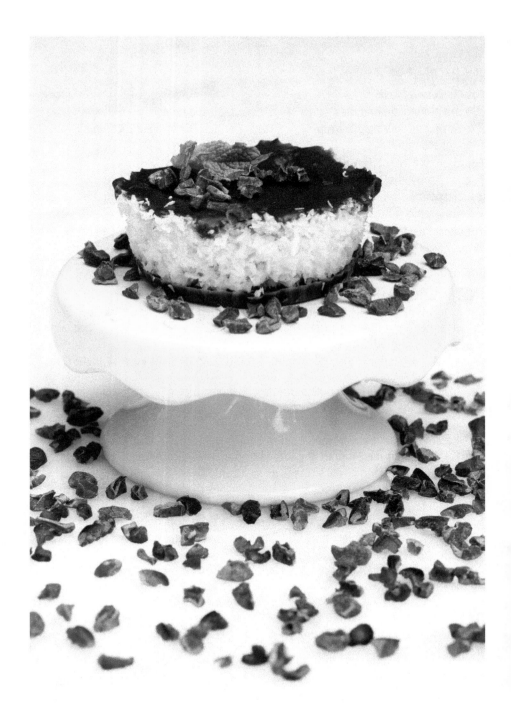

Peppermint Patties

INGREDIENTS:

Chocolate:
8 tablespoons coconut oil, melted
4 tablespoons raw cacao powder or cocoa powder
4 tablespoons maple syrup   A few grains of salt

Peppermint Patty:
2 cups unsweetened shredded coconut
½ teaspoon (food-grade) peppermint essential oil or
1 teaspoon of peppermint extract
4 tablespoons maple syrup   6 tablespoons hot water

INSTRUCTIONS:
1. Line a 12-count muffin tin with paper or silicone muffin liners.
2. In a food processor, blend all ingredients together for the chocolate. (It will be on the liquid side of textures.)
3. Pour chocolate into the base of each muffin tin, just covering the bottom, and leaving about ⅓ of the chocolate in the mixing bowl.
4. Allow chocolate in the muffin tin to cool in the freezer.
5. In a food processor, add the coconut, peppermint, maple syrup, and hot water. Blend until everything is well combined.
6. Remove chocolate from the freezer.
7. Add a tablespoon (or so) of coconut mixture on top of the chocolate, pressing gently.
8. Drizzle remaining chocolate over the tops of the coconut.
9. Cool in the freezer for approximately 10-20 minutes.
10. Remove liner and ENJOY!
Note: Best if stored in the freezer.
Serves approximately 12

Traditional Peppermint Patties Ingredients
(Inflammatory Foods Highlighted in Bold Italics)
Sugar, Corn Syrup, Semi-Sweet Chocolate (Chocolate, ***Sugar,*** Cocoa, ***Milk Fat,*** Cocoa Butter, ***Soy*** Lecithin, ***Emulsifier,*** Vanilla, ***Artificial Flavor***) ***Invert Sugar,*** Egg Whites, Oil of Peppermint, ***Milk***

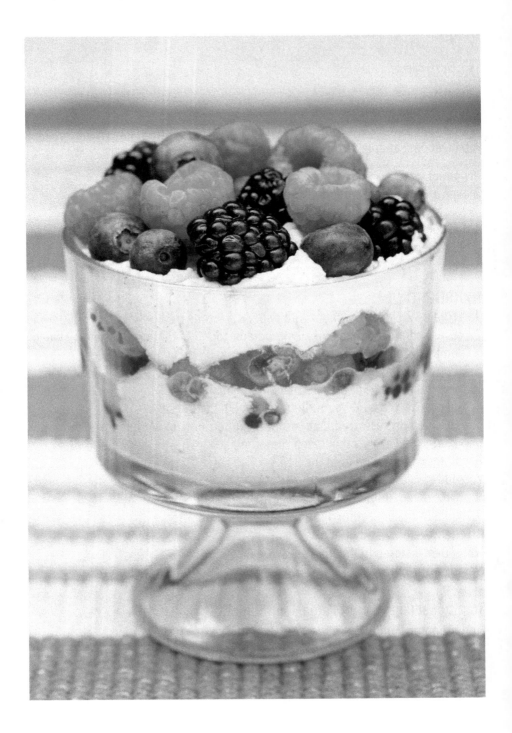

Coconut Whipped Cream with Berries

INGREDIENTS:
2 cans of full fat coconut milk (cream only), chilled overnight
3-4 tablespoons pure maple syrup
3 teaspoons vanilla extract
½ teaspoon almond extract
½-1 teaspoon pumpkin pie spice
Fresh organic berries to top

INSTRUCTIONS:
1. To get started, you will want to chill your cans of coconut milk in the fridge for at least 6 hours, preferably overnight. When you remove the chilled can, be careful not to shake it.
2. Carefully open the can of coconut milk and scoop the thickened cream into a bowl, leaving behind the liquid coconut water.
3. Add the pure maple syrup, vanilla extract, almond extract, and pumpkin pie spice to the heavy coconut cream. Mix thoroughly with a hand mixer – will take 3-5 minutes for peaks to form.
4. Serve immediately or keep in the refrigerator to allow it to set more.

Serves 6-8

Traditional Whipped Cream Ingredients
(Inflammatory Foods Highlighted in Bold Italics)
Heavy Cream, Sugar, Nonfat Milk, Artificial Flavor, Sorbitan Monostearate, Carrageenan, Mixed Tocopherols

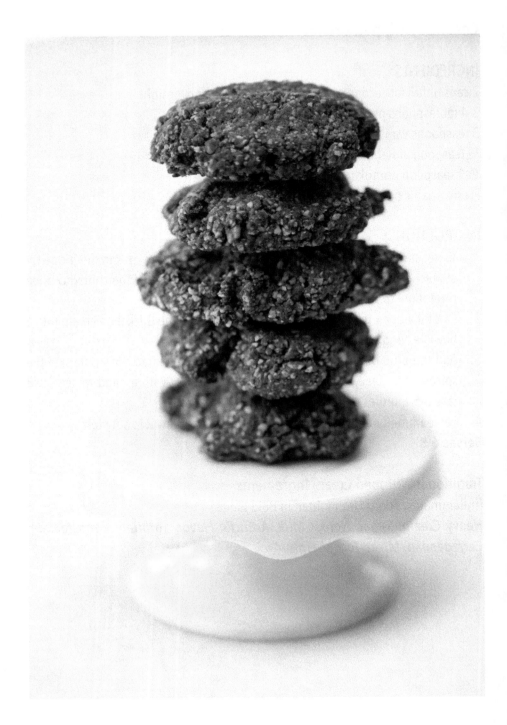

Chocolate Hazelnut Cookies

INGREDIENTS:

1 cup whole raw hazelnuts or pecans

⅓ cup whole raw almonds

¼ cup coconut flour

¼ cup raw cacao powder

½ teaspoon baking soda

⅛ teaspoon sea salt

2 dried Medjool dates (pitted)

¼ cup softened virgin coconut oil

½ teaspoon vanilla extract

1-2 teaspoons raw honey

INSTRUCTIONS:

1. Preheat oven to 350 degrees.
2. In a food processor, grind hazelnuts or pecans until coarse.
3. Add almonds and blend until nuts release just a bit of oil.
4. Add coconut flour and pulse.
5. Add cocoa powder and pulse.
6. Add baking soda and sea salt. Pulse again; the mixture should feel like fine flour.
7. Transfer the dry ingredients to a bowl. Clean out food processor.
8. In empty food processor, add dates, coconut oil, raw honey and vanilla. Pulse until well incorporated.
9. Mix together the dry and wet mixtures.
10. Form small balls and gently press down into a cookie sheet lined with parchment paper.
11. Bake at 350 degrees for 8-10 minutes.

Serves 16-20

Traditional Chocolate Hazelnut Cookie Ingredients

(Inflammatory Foods Highlighted in Bold Italics)

Hazelnuts, ***All Purpose Flour,*** Unsweetened Cocoa Powder, Baking Powder, ***Salt, Butter, Sugar,*** Egg, ***Dark Rum***

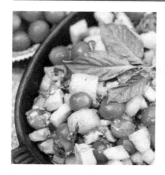
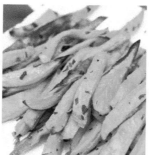
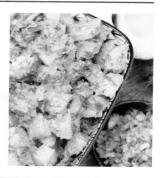

Food Swap

Recipes for Sides

Recipes Free Of: Processed Sugar, Wheat, Cow Dairy, Inflammatory Oils & GMOs

(Be sure to check out the traditional inflammatory foods at the bottom of each recipe, so you can continue to learn what is inflammatory and how to swap those out for non-inflammatory ingredients.)

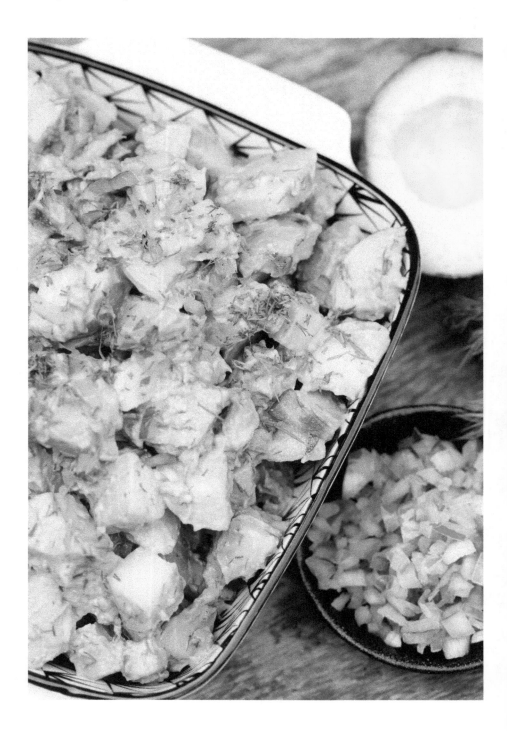

Creamy Avocado Potato Salad

INGREDIENTS:

3 pounds Yukon gold potatoes
4 tablespoons Dijon mustard
4 tablespoons fresh dill, chopped
2 teaspoons fresh lemon juice
Black pepper, to taste

2 ripe avocados
4 tablespoons diced red onion
1 cup cucumber, chopped
¼ teaspoon salt, or to taste

INSTRUCTIONS:

1. Scrub the potatoes well, then chop into 1-inch cubes. Add potatoes to a pot of water and boil for about 10 minutes, or until the potato chunks are for tender. (Be careful not to overcook.)

2. While the potatoes are cooking, combine the avocado, Dijon mustard, red onion, cucumber, dill, lemon juice, and salt in a medium bowl and mash with a fork. This mixture will be acidic-tasting until mixed with the potatoes, but feel free to adjust any flavors to suit your taste.

3. Allow the steamed potatoes to cool for at least 20 minutes (preferably in the fridge to speed things up) then gradually add the potatoes to the creamy avocado sauce, mixing gently to coat well.

4. Allow the potatoes to marinate in the fridge for at least an hour, so the potato salad can completely cool. Serve chilled.

Serves 6

Traditional Potato Salad Ingredients
(Inflammatory Foods Highlighted in Bold Italics)
Potatoes, ***Mayonnaise,*** Vinegar, ***Salt, Sugar,*** Black Pepper, Onion, Egg

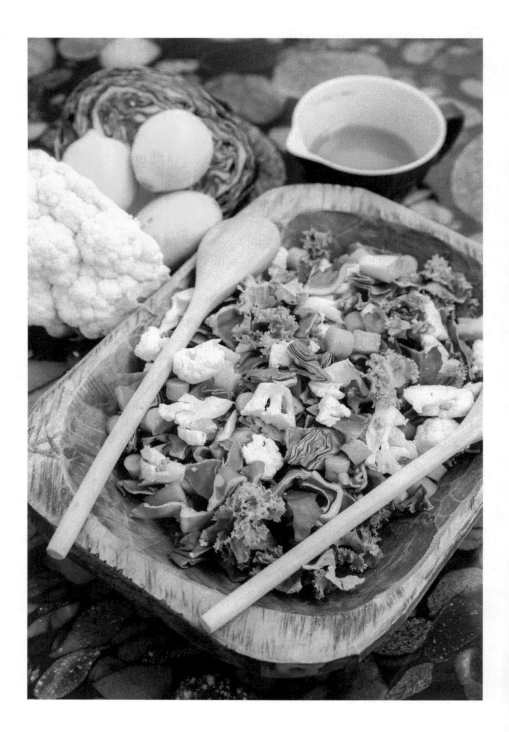

Sweet Chop Salad

INGREDIENTS:
1 bunch of organic kale
1 organic apple
½ head organic purple cabbage
4 large organic carrots
½ head organic cauliflower
⅓ cup of Cara Cara Orange Vanilla White Balsamic vinegar from www.genesis-kitchen.com
⅓ cup Blood Orange Olive Oil from www.genesis-kitchen.com

INSTRUCTIONS:
1. Chop up all of the vegetables into bite sized pieces. (You can add broccoli, chard and any other vegetable that do not get soggy when marinating in dressing.)
2. Mix vegetables with oil and vinegar.
3. Allow the vegetables to marinate in the dressing for at least 30 minutes.
4. The salad will keep for most of the week in the refrigerator.

Serves 10

Note: Genesis Kitchen makes EVOO and vinegars that are of the highest qualities without processed sugars or added inflammatory ingredients. They are also the most affordable that I am aware of, for the quality. With that said, it is not necessary to purchase from them, just an option.

Traditional Chop Salad Ingredients
(Inflammatory Foods Highlighted in Bold Italics)
Vegetables, *Canola Oil,* Vinegar, *Herbs, Sugar, Salt*

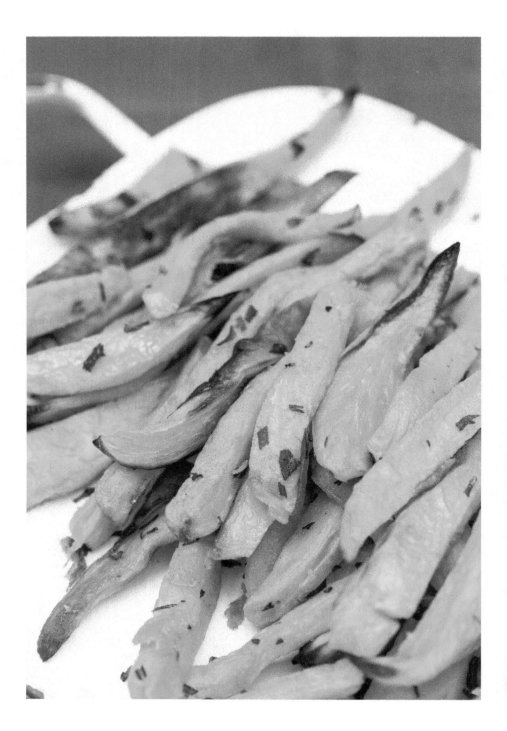

Roasted Yam Fries

INGREDIENTS:
5 large sweet potatoes
¼ cup extra virgin olive oil
2 tablespoons dried rosemary
1 ½ teaspoons sea salt
1 teaspoon ground garlic

INSTRUCTIONS:
1. Preheat oven to 450 degrees. (For more crispiness, preheat to 500 degrees and then turn down once sweet potatoes go in the oven.)
2. Cut the potatoes in long strips.
3. Put the sweet potatoes into a large bowl and add the olive oil; mix well.
4. Sprinkle with salt, rosemary, and spices of your choice. It is fun to play around with cayenne, cinnamon, etc.
5. Use your hands to mix well, so all pieces are covered with oil and spices.
6. Spread the pieces out in a single layer on a baking sheet.
7. Bake for a total of 25 to 30 minutes. After the first 15 minutes, remove the baking sheet from the oven and turn all the pieces over. Return to the oven to bake for another 10 to 15 minutes, or until they are well browned.
8. Let cool for 5 minutes before serving.

Makes two large cookie sheets worth of fries

Traditional Fast Food French Fry Ingredients
(Inflammatory Foods Highlighted in Bold Italics)
Potatoes, ***Vegetable Oil, Canola Oil, Soybean Oil, Hydrogenated Soybean Oil, Natural Beef Flavor, Citric Acid, Dextrose, Sodium Acid Prophosphate, Salt***

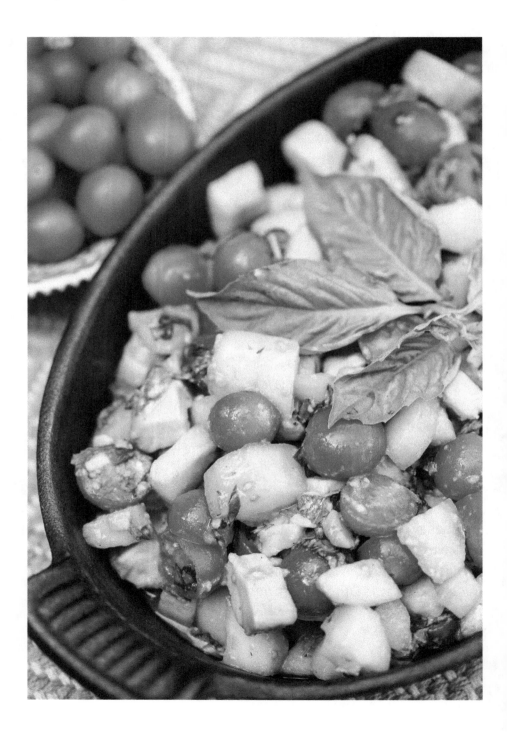

Cucumber, Avocado, & Tomato Salad

INGREDIENTS:
2 avocados
1 pint of cherry tomatoes
2 cucumbers, peeled and chopped into small pieces
½ cup extra virgin olive oil (I love the basil infused EVOO at www.genesis-kitchen.com)
2 tablespoons balsamic vinegar (no sugar added)
2 teaspoons chopped fresh basil
Sea salt

INSTRUCTIONS:
1. Cube and slice avocados and cucumber.
2. Halve the tomatoes.
3. Mix extra virgin olive oil, balsamic vinegar, and basil in a separate bowl.
4. Toss olive oil and herbs into the salad.
5. Add sea salt to taste.

Serves 6

Traditional Cucumber, Avocado, & Tomato Salad Ingredients
(Inflammatory Foods Highlighted in Bold Italics)
Avocado, Tomato, Cucumber, and Extra Virgin Olive Oil. No inflammatory ingredients here.

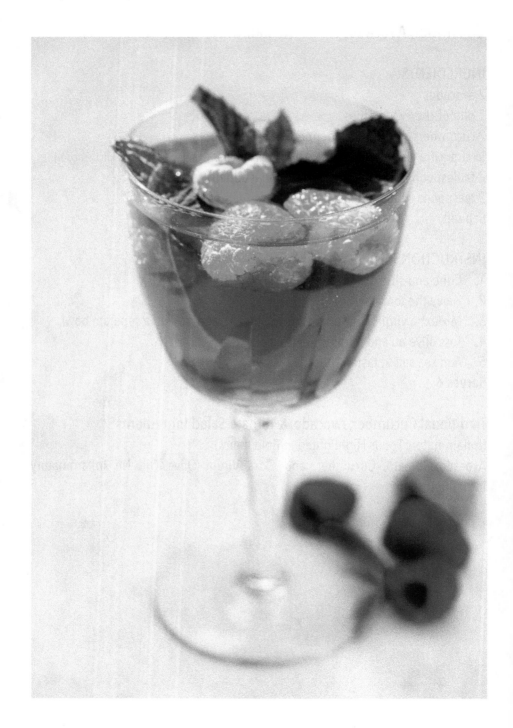

My Favorite Mocktail

Harmless Harvest Raw Coconut Water
garnished with organic raspberries and a mint sprig.
Served in grandma's crystal wine glass.

Further Reading

Sugar Has 56 Names, by Dr. Robert Lustig, MD

The Real Truth About Sugar, by Dr. Robert Lustig, MD

Pure, White, and Deadly, by John Yudkin

Blood Sugar Solution, by Mark Hyman, MD

Eat Fat, Get Thin, by Mark Hyman, MD

Real Food Diet Cookbook, by Dr. Josh Axe

Hidden Secrets To Curing Your Chronic Disease, by Dr. Jason West

Healthy Aging, by Andrew Weil, MD

Acknowledgments

My heart is overflowing with gratitude for every single person who helped to make this book come to fruition, which is a long list of people. First, to my family. Mom and dad, words do not exist for the infinite support, love, and believe-in-me power you have wrapped me in. Thank you for always seeing me both as who I am, and as who I have the potential to be. I love you. Brock, you encouraged me to jump all in and write this book even when I was unsure of my ability to do so. You have pulled off many late nights and weekends playing with Tosh and Chloe so I can meet my deadlines. It is not only your encouragement, but your daily and hourly support helping our household stay together that has made the biggest difference. I am deeply grateful. XO

And to Tosh and Chloe. Had it not been for you showing up in this life, teaching me the power of inflammation along with the healing that can be accomplished through foods, I would likely be living a very different life. Thank you for being my teachers, now and forever.

To Angela Lauria, who saw my vision, believed in my ability to help others around the world, and chose me to share this message in this book – thank you. Not only am I deeply grateful to have you as my coach, but your ability to help me grow and transform my world in major ways is a gift that will be with me forever.

Eeva Pregitzer, Aaron Kraft, and Nicole Robertson, your friendship has helped to bring me through some of my darkest times. Thank you for always accepting me, even when I struggled to do so for myself. I treasure each of you.

Jamye Chrisman, you showed up ready to take photos and make my food come to life – even on a crazy deadline. Thank you for believing in this work and for your desire to help spread health and joy around the world.

Had it not been for the following people who volunteered their time to cook recipes and style food for our photo shoot, this book would be lacking color and life. Barb Huhn, Lenor Taggart, Kathy Bressler, Tena Looney, Claire Perrin, Emily Bain, Penny McBride, David Bressler, Lauren Harris, and Nicole Robertson, thank you for your tremendous help in donating over 60 hours of combined time to make this book a tremendous success. For everyone else who contributed to this book, but whose name I did not mention, know that I give gratitude to you each day.

To the Morgan James Publishing team: Special thanks to David Hancock, CEO & Founder for believing in me and my message. To my Author Relations Manager, Bonnie Rauch, thanks for making the process seamless and easy. Many more thanks to everyone else, but especially Jim Howard, Bethany Marshall, and Nickcole Watkins.

Last, but certainly not least, the gratitude I have for my current, past and future clients goes far beyond business. Thank you for trusting me, for showing your vulnerable side, and for being open to take each step down this path of unbelievable health, joy, and enlightenment. Because of you, I show up for myself in bigger and better ways each day and together we get to be the change we wish to see in the world. I thank you.

About the Author

Jenny Carr is an anti-inflammatory health coach, a motivational speaker, a mom and an international best selling author. She went through a near death experience due to chronic illness and survived, by walking her talk in regards to anti-inflammatory living. While she was passionate about anti-inflammatory eating before, this near death experienced inspired her to share as much as she can with the world, to help others heal. She specializes in helping people reverse chronic 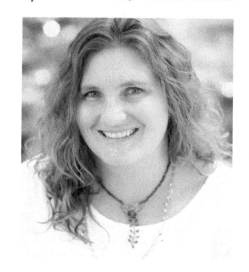 symptoms through anti-inflammatory eating without feeling deprived or overwhelmed.

Jenny has spent that last 6 years helping hundreds of people identify what is inflaming them and how to swap out those foods for options that do not inflame, but still satisfy. She knows first hand what life as a busy parent looks like and she is committed to making anti-inflammatory eating a reality for all people, no matter their lifestyle. Jenny is passionate about helping people melt away inflammation and living a life free to do what they enjoy without complications from health ailments.

Part anti-inflammatory health coach and part life-coach, Jenny intertwines these two coaching modalities to help people make lasting changes in their life. She holds a masters in education, is a certified personal trainer and certified health coach and holds extensive training in alternative and integrative nutrition, childhood and adolescent nutrition as well as a fitness and nutrition specialist. Jenny's favorite part of her work is helping to take her clients from dis-ease and degeneration to empowerment, health and vibrancy.

Jenny currently lives in Jackson Hole, WY. She loves spending time with her family and enjoys whipping up new recipes, connecting to the great outdoors and furthering her own self-growth.

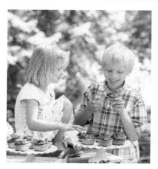 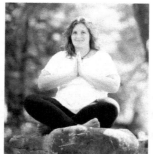 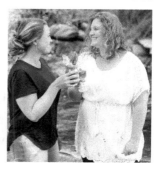

Thank You

How To Travel & Follow Anti-Inflammatory Eating

*Learn how to follow an anti-inflammatory diet while traveling,
AND enjoy your food so you can feel great.*

Thank you for reading *Peace of Cake!* One of the biggest obstacles I often hear about from clients following an anti-inflammatory diet is maintaining healthy eating habits while on the road. Whether you are an avid business traveler or love traveling for personal enjoyment, I've got a few tips to keep you feeling great while enjoying your time away from home. Simply go to www.peaceofcakebook.com and sign up for the FREE 3-part video series. ***Fun Fact*** – even if you are not a big traveler, these tips will help you move through days when food prep falls low on the totem pole, but you still need to maintain anti-inflammatory eating.

With love,
Jenny Carr

P.S. *Peace of Cake* is the culmination of my dream come true. I've always wanted to write a book that makes a difference in the world and I would ***love*** to know how it has helped you in your life. Feel free to email me (jenny@jennycarrhealth.com) or comment on Facebook at Jenny Carr Health to share your story.

To learn more about Jenny's next book, *The Clean Eating Kid*, visit her website:

www.jennycarrhealth.com

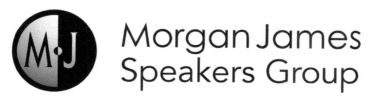

Morgan James
Speakers Group

We connect Morgan James published authors with live and online events and audiences who will benefit from their expertise.

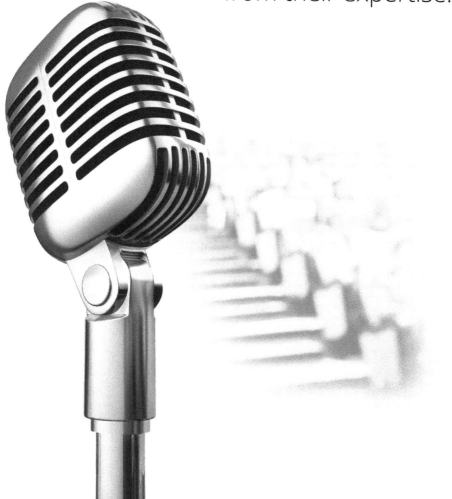

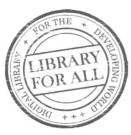

CPSIA information can be obtained
at www.ICGtesting.com
Printed in the USA
BVHW092345111118
532816BV00003B/14/P